NOURISH YOUR WAY TO A HEALTHY WEIGHT: EMBRACE FOOD, TRUST YOUR BODY, AND ACHIEVE LASTING RESULTS

BY

ELLA F. MILLER

Disclaimer

Acknowledgment

Nourish Your Way to a Healthy Weight is a great and magnificent source of blessing and I am grateful to those who have made this experience feasible.

To my family for their ongoing help and faith in my task.

To medical specialists for important expertise.

To my persecutors and allies for driving my substance

To local invention, to push the bounds

For nature, this is proof of connectedness, revelation and progress for this revolutionary voyage.

As we embrace life and regular weight reduction, our routes are established by associations and intelligence. Thank you to everyone who took part in our trip.

Thankfully,

Ella F. Miller

Table of Content

Create a long-term plan for sustainable results: Your Roadmap to Sustainable Wellness

Final thoughts: a road map for sustainable well-being
Player Digest

Book Review

"Nourish Your Way to a Healthy Weight" is a revolutionary technique for natural weight loss. It modifies your attitude towards weight reduction by concentrating on balance and mindfulness.

This book invites you to listen to your body and make mindful food choices. It also emphasizes the benefits of enjoying your favorite foods in moderation.

Staying active is vital, and the book contains practical techniques to incorporate pleasant exercise into your daily life.

"Healthy Habits for Life" stresses sustainable lifestyle improvements, such as stress management and sleep, for long-term success.

In conclusion, "Nourish Your Way to a Healthy Weight" gives a straightforward and holistic approach to weight loss. If you want to achieve natural weight loss with balance and mindfulness, this book is a must-read.

About The Author

Ella F. Miller is a dedicated supporter of holistic health and well-being. With considerable education and a belief in balance, she brings a wealth of skills to "Nourish Your Way to a Healthy Weight".

Ella F. Miller has effectively assisted clients on their weight loss journeys, emphasizing self-awareness and self-compassion.

Her language is empathetic and transparent, making it easier to understand complicated health conditions. She's committed to giving a transforming approach to holistic health, enabling individuals to live happier, healthier lives.

Ella F. Miller continues to support conscious life and natural weight loss, urging individuals to appreciate life fully.

Introduction

In a world faced with countless diets, fashion, and weight loss plans, "Nourish Your Way to a Healthy Weight" stands out as a light of clarity and authenticity. The adventure that you are going to start is not just to shed those unwanted pounds. It is a deep study of the complex connection between your body and the nutrients it desires. Here, you will discover the transformative power of accepting food as more than just fuel but as a vital source of health, healing, and self-discovery.

In the following pages, we will clarify popular myths and misunderstandings about weight reduction and reveal the science behind sustainable, lasting results. You will learn to trust the inner wisdom of your body, allowing it to guide you towards your optimal weight naturally. There are no more strict rules or deprivations. Instead, you will gain an intuitive understanding of what your body really needs to thrive.

This book is not just another guide. It is a useful companion on your journey to health and well-being. We have combined the latest research and knowledge from nutritionists, psychologists, and health lovers to present you with an integrated, evidence-based approach. You will gain a deeper knowledge of the complex interaction between food, emotions, and behavior, helping you make informed choices that match your goals.

But this book is not just about science and facts. It is also a celebration of real success stories by those who have walked this journey before you. Their stories, challenges, and achievements will inspire and guide you, reminding you that sustainable transformation is not only possible but also profoundly satisfactory.

We ask you to open your hearts and minds as you turn every page, ready to adopt a healthier lifestyle that transcends numbers on a scale. "Nourish Your Way to a Healthy Weight" is your invitation to a journey of self-discovery, self-care, and self-power. Together, we will uncover the secrets to achieving a healthier, happier self — not just for a season, but for a lifetime. So, let's dive and start this wonderful adventure towards lasting health and energy.

Chapter 1: Awakening to the Magic of Food

Welcome to the first part of our wonderful journey, where we go on a voyage into the captivating realm of nutrition. In these pages, we will explore the idea that food is not just a fuel; it is a powerful enchantress that holds the key to unlocking the actual potential of your body. Prepare for a fascinating voyage packed with inspiration, intuition, and actionable insight as we create the foundations for your transformation to lasting well-being.

Our objective in this chapter is to clarify common myths and misconceptions that often impede our understanding of food. We hope to provide you with a different perspective, one that shows how each meal-time decision is a step towards a healthier and more energetic version of yourself.

The knowledge you will obtain here will serve as a foundation on which we will build in the upcoming chapters. Our approach is comprehensive, addressing not just the physical component of health but also the profound link between diet, emotions, and psychology. You will discover that food is not simply what you consume; it is also the relationship you create with food.

Through this chapter, you will be introduced to the true experiences of individuals who have harnessed the extraordinary power of diet to redefine their lives. These stories are not simply narrative but deeply inspiring, revealing that the journey to a healthier weight is not a solo battle but a collaborative triumph of self-discovery and endurance.

But let's go deeper. Beyond dispelling myths and exchanging tales, we will learn the science behind nutrition. You will learn about how the food you eat affects your body at a cellular level, from energy metabolism to hormone control. This understanding will enable you to make informed decisions that match your health and well-being goals.

So, as we begin this amazing voyage, we invite you to open your heart and mind. It is time to awaken to the charm of eating, where food transcends mere food and becomes a powerful instrument of personal development. Together, we will uncover the dormant potential inside you and prepare for a life full of health, happiness, and vigor. Prepare to embrace the magic of eating like never before.

Follow Through and Let's Explore Linda's Weight Loss Journey

In a bustling city, in the midst of the daily bustle and the clamor of life, lived a woman named Linda. She had always been recognized for her lively personality and contagious laughter, but under her pleasant look, Linda carried a burden that had developed over time.

One evening, while preparing for the meeting with a friend, Linda stood in front of the mirror in her room, inspecting her appearance with a mixture of annoyance and despair. The clothes she admired now felt like garments of self-doubt. The picture that looked at her was not the one she was proud of.

She blew, understanding that her weight had not only taken a knock on her confidence but had also begun to impair her health. The rising of the stairs made her breathless, and her doctor had gently advised her of the significance of making a change for her well-being.

Linda, like so many others who have found themselves at a similar junction, felt that she needed a change. It was not about conforming to a particular size of clothes or adhering to society's ideals of beauty. It was about restoring her health and vitality and feeling comfortable in her own flesh.

One day, while perusing the internet, Linda came upon a book that would change the path of her journey. The book was called "Nourish Your Way to a Healthy Weight." The phrase alone drew her because it promised something different— something beyond the rigid diets and rapid solutions she had encountered before.

With a sense of hope mingled with skepticism, Linda decided to read it. Little did she know that this book was going to become her guiding light, illuminating the path of transformation that lay before her.

As Linda plunges into the pages of the book, she starts on a journey of self-discovery. She understood the value of sustaining her body with excellent nutrients, knowing the genuine purpose of eating. It wasn't about restricting or tracking calories; it was about choosing choices that valued your well-being.

With every chapter she devours, Linda feels a change in herself. She came to comprehend that her mission was not just to lose pounds; it was to adopt a new way of life. She has learned to eat mindfully, to listen to her body's signs, to taste every bite, and to be present in the moment.

The book also introduced Linda to the concept of faith in the knowledge of her body. She discovered that her body had its own way of informing her when he was hungry and when he had enough. It was a breakthrough—the one that allowed her to let up the weighty rules and constraints that had plummeted her prior weight-loss endeavors.

With improved information and a sense of empowerment, Linda began to make changes in her life. She began to experiment with different foods, to add more fruit and vegetables to her diet, and to enjoy the flavors of authentic and unprocessed dishes. It was a gradual process, filled with minor victories and a rising sense of self-confidence.

Linda's quest had begun, and although the route before her was uncertain, she felt a flush of hope. She knew that this time, it was not just about achieving a destination but about embracing the journey itself. It was about feeding his body, following his instincts, and, most importantly, learning to love each other along the way.

And so, with every page and every meal that valued her body, Linda took her first steps on the path to a healthier, happier, and more fulfilled life.

Understanding The True Meaning of Nourishment

In our fast and modern society, the concept of eating is sometimes too simplified, reduced to simply calorie counting, or guided by the newest food trends. However, if we are to embark on a meaningful road towards a healthier weight and a better life, it is vital to cut the layers and genuinely comprehend the deep, multidimensional role of food.

Nutrition spans much more than the food we eat; it embraces all the components that sustain and nurture our bodies, brains, and souls. Let's dig deeper into each dimension of this concept:

Physical Nutrition: Physical nutrition is centered on giving your body the resources it needs to perform successfully. It's about choosing foods that not only pleasure your taste senses but also give you the vitamins, minerals, and energy needed for your body's everyday responsibilities. Think about feeding your body as well as filling your automobile with the highest grade of gasoline—you make sure it works smoothly and efficiently.

Emotional Food: Our emotions play a key part in our engagement with food. Emotionally feeding means knowing that food can offer comfort, joy, and celebration in our lives. However, it also requires being sensitive about how we use food to cope with stress or conceal feelings. Understanding the emotional components of eating helps us make healthier decisions while enjoying the pleasure that food may provide.

Psychological Food: The way we see food, our self-image, and our self-esteem all influence our eating patterns. Psychological nutrition entails creating a healthy relationship with food and cultivating self-compassion. It is about releasing ourselves from the shame frequently linked with abandonment and building a balanced and sustainable approach to food.

Social Nutrition: Food has exceptional potential to bring people together and develop bonds and collaborations. Sharing meals with loved ones offers a sense of belonging and enjoyment. Social nutrition reminds us that food is not just a question of nutrients; it is a tool for building expensive experiences and forging ties.

Spiritual Care: At a deeper level, caring can be spiritual. It is about finding purpose, meaning, and complete awareness in your dietary choices. It could involve behaviors such as dining thoughtfully when you taste every piece and connect with the spirit of food. Spiritual food may provide a wonderful sense of satisfaction and awareness to your eating experience, letting you recognize the interconnection of all life.

Understanding the true meaning of nutrition is the cornerstone of your route to a healthier weight and a more balanced existence. It is about recognizing that eating is not a single notion but a full, multidimensional approach to well-being. By embracing food in all its dimensions, you can unlock the capacity to make enduring gains, not only in your body but in your total well-being.

So, let's travel together on this trip of enlightenment, where we will explore the magic of food from all sides, acquiring crucial ideas and techniques to nourish our bodies, our brains, and our thoughts for a healthy and happy existence.

Developing A Positive Relationship with Food

In a world often focused on diets and quick solutions, the idea of developing a joyful relationship with food could seem like a distant dream. However, it is not simply an ideal; it is a very practical and achievable aim that may enhance your relationship to eating, your overall health, and your sense of well-being.

So, let's plunge in and learn the approaches to developing a pleasurable and caring connection with food:

Eliminate food Guilt: One of the first steps towards building a positive connection with food is to eliminate the food blame. Realize that there is no such thing as "good" or "bad" food. Food is not a moral compass. Allowing frequent sweets or indulgences without feeling guilty is the key. In fact, this is part of a balanced approach to nutrition. Instead of punishing

Practice Attentive Eating: Eating attentively involves being totally present during your meals. It's about enjoying every bite, experiencing the flavors and textures, and paying attention to your body's indicators of hunger and satiety. When you intentionally eat, you are less inclined to exaggerate, and you build a deeper relationship with the food you consume. Try to put away distractions like your phone or TV during meals and appreciate the moment.

Restrictive Diets: Restraining diets frequently do more harm than good. They can build an excessive attachment to food and lead to cycles of restriction and overindulgence. Instead, focus on healthy, sustainable eating practices that you can maintain in the long term. Think of food as fuel for your body rather than as something to fear or control.

Listen to Your Body: Your body is an expert advisor when it comes to nutrition. Learn to conform to your indicators of hunger and satiety. When you're hungry, eat, and when you've eaten enough stop. Trust your body's messages; it knows what it needs. This can mean eating smaller, more regular meals or enjoying larger, less frequent meals; everyone's body is unique.

Celebrate Food: Nutrition is not just nutrition; it is a source of pleasure and happiness. Celebrate the eating experience by discovering new sensations, experiencing other cuisines, and sharing meals with loved ones. When you consider food as a source of delight, it becomes easy to build a positive relationship with it. Consider cooking and experimenting with recipes as a way to connect with the creative and joyous side of eating.

Forgive Yourself: We all have instances when we drink more than we expected or make less than optimal decisions. It is vital to practice self-compassion and forgive yourself for these situations. Remember that a single meal or snack does not define your overall eating habits. Instead of focusing on a perceived "error," focus on making the following alternative a healthier option without judgment or guilt.

Search for Support: Establishing a good connection with food can be tough, especially if you have a history of diet or chaotic eating. Consider seeking treatment from a licensed dietician or a therapist who specializes in intuitive eating disorders. They can provide direction and resources to support you on your road and deal with any underlying emotional or psychological problems that can influence your relationship with food.

Remember, developing a healthy connection with food is a process, and it's good to do it one step at a time. The goal is to establish a sustainable, pleasurable, and nutritious approach to eating that supports your health and well-being. By exercising compassion for yourself and recognizing food as a source of food and pleasure, you can shift your relationship by feeding it for the better, eventually leading to a healthier and happier you. It is about building a lifelong partnership with food that serves as a source of strength, joy, and subsistence for your body and soul.

Embrace A Balanced Approach to Nutrition

In a world inundated with extreme food fads and contradicting nutritional advice, the idea of having a balanced approach to diet is like locating a compass in the middle of a cyclone. It is not an issue of harsh restrictions or self-denial; on the contrary, it is a way to a pleasant and permanent relationship with food. Let's unfold this concept further and figure out how to make a balanced diet a natural and pleasurable part of your daily life.

Get rid of the thinking of nothing or nothing: A balanced approach to food begins by discarding the perspective of nothing or nothing. Understand that perfection in your diet is a myth, and some indulgences are not only acceptable but wonderful. It's about finding a medium ground where you may enjoy your favorite indulgences without guilt while keeping an emphasis on feeding your body with nutrient-rich foods. This balance provides flexibility and pleasure in your eating habits.

Prioritize Complete and Nutrient-rich Foods: To develop a balanced diet, focus on incorporating a full range of nutrient-rich foods into your diet. These are foods that provide vitamins, minerals, fiber, and other necessary nutrients. Think of a rainbow of colorful fruits and vegetables, lean forms of protein like chicken, fish, or herbal alternatives, nutritious grains like quinoa or brown rice, and healthy fats from sources like avocados and almonds. These foods not only sustain your body but also fill your palette with a diverse tapestry of flavors and textures.

Portion Control: Paying attention to portion proportions is vital for a balanced diet. It is easy to eat too much when portions are excessively large, even if you consume nutritious items. Using smaller dishes, weighing your meals, and paying attention to portion sizes will help you maintain balance and reduce overindulgence. Remember, enjoying modest amounts of your favorite foods can be as delightful as larger portions.

Listen to Your Body: Your body is an amazing guide when it comes to eating. Beware of symptoms of hunger and satiety. Eat when you are hungry, and quit when you're content. This natural method of feeding helps you maintain balance without the need for stringent rules or external signs. It's about building trust in the knowledge of your body and obeying its clues.

Practice Meal Planning: Planning your meals and snacks in advance will help you make balanced choices throughout the day. Include a combination of food groups in each meal, such as proteins, vegetables, and whole grains, to ensure you obtain a well-rounded nutritional intake. Meal planning not only supports a balanced diet but also simplifies your everyday dietary decisions.

Enjoy the Treatments Carefully: It is quite beneficial to enjoy the traits and decadent foods of a balanced diet. The thing is to do it carefully. Savor each bite, and be present in the moment. A healthy diet boosts your pleasure and helps prevent overindulgence by allowing you to completely enjoy the flavors and textures of your favorite dishes. This strategy allows you to find fulfillment in fewer servings and eliminates the impulse to overconsume.

Stay Hydrated: Sometimes thirst can be concealed like hunger, leading to excessive snacks or overeating. Be sure to hydrate yourself with water throughout the day. Staying hydrated might help you make more balanced eating choices by dealing with true hunger rather than thirst.

Learn More about Nutrition: Knowledge is power when it comes to a balanced diet. Educate yourself on nutrition to make informed choices. Understand the relevance of different nutrients for your health and well-being. This awareness helps you make balanced choices that match your goals, whether they involve weight management, greater energy levels, or overall well-being.

Search Variety: Eating a variety of foods not only keeps your meals interesting but also guarantees you acquire a diverse range of nutrients. Experiment with different cuisines, flavors, and ingredients to keep your taste buds intrigued and appreciate the wide range of nutrients that different foods supply. The variety also eliminates nutritional monotony, which encourages commitment to a long-term balanced diet.

Practice Self-Compassion: Finally, remember that a balanced approach to food also includes self-compassion. If you have a day when your decisions do not perfectly fit your goals, do not fight. Instead, accept that it's a part of life and focus on a balanced diet for your next meal or snack. Self-compassion is a powerful method that fosters a healthy relationship with food by minimizing guilt and developing a sense of self-care and self-acceptance.

Taking a balanced approach to nutrition is not a matter of perfection; it is about finding harmony and sustainability in your relationship with food. It is a voyage of self-discovery and self-care where you feed your body while simultaneously enjoying the delights of food. By renouncing severe dieting and adopting moderation and full consciousness,

Chapter 2: Trusting Your Body's Wisdom

Welcome to chapter 2 of our journey of transformation, where we take a deeper look at the key concept of faith in the understanding of your body. In a world that often bombards us with external rules and expectations about what, when, and how much to eat, this chapter is a good reminder that your body holds natural wisdom when it comes to eating.

Understanding The True Significance of Food

Why am I overweight?

Before commencing the journey of weight management and self-discovery, it is necessary to know that being overweight or struggling with excess weight is not a simple equation with a single cause. Rather, it is a complex problem influenced by many elements that might vary widely from person to person. Considering these factors can shed light on why some people may be overweight. Here are numerous key reasons:

1. Diet and Dietary Habits: One of the most evident reasons that lead to becoming overweight is dietary choices and habits. Eating a high-calorie diet, processed foods, sugary drinks, and excessive amounts might lead to weight gain over time. Unhealthy eating patterns, such as emotional eating or mindless nibbling, can make the situation even worse.

2. Sedentary Lifestyle: Our modern, technology-driven lives typically prefer a sedentary lifestyle. Spending longer hours sitting in workplaces, in front of screens, or in cars can drastically diminish levels of physical exercise. Lack of regular exercise can contribute to weight gain and the loss of muscular mass.

3. Genetic: Genetics has a part in establishing an individual's predisposition to weight gain and obesity. Certain genetic characteristics can influence metabolism, hunger management, and the way the body stores and consumes fat. While genetics may predispose someone to weight gain, they do not decide their fate; lifestyle choices always play a critical role.

4. Psychological Factors: Emotional and psychological reasons might sometimes be at the heart of weight troubles. Stress, sadness, anxiety, trauma, and other emotional challenges can lead to overeating or the adoption of improper management practices. Emotional eating, in particular, is a common component of being overweight.

5. Medical Conditions: Certain hormonal diseases and imbalances may contribute to weight gain. Conditions such as polycystic ovary syndrome (PCOS), thyroid issues, and insulin resistance can change metabolism and appetite regulation, making it tougher to maintain a healthy weight.

6. Medications: Some drugs, especially particular antidepressants, antipsychotics, and corticosteroids, are known to be connected to weight gain as a side effect. These medicines can change appetite and metabolism, making it tougher to manage weight.

7. Socio-economic Factors: Socio-economic variables could potentially play a part in weight management. Limited access to nutritious meals owing to budgetary restrictions, living in food deserts, or a lack of understanding of healthy eating can lead to weight problems.

8. Lack of Knowledge and Information: Sometimes people may be overweight simply because of a lack of understanding about good eating habits and the necessity for physical activity. This lack of information may be the result of insufficient access to educational resources or cultural pressures that emphasize other parts of life.

9. Environmental Factors: The environment in which a person lives might influence weight management. A community with limited opportunities for physical activity, a proliferation of fast-food restaurants, and a lack of safe outdoor spaces could make it more difficult to maintain a healthy weight.

10. Social and Cultural Influences: Social and cultural elements might alter our eating habits and our beliefs about body image. Pressure to comply with certain beauty standards or cultural traditions that revolve around food can contribute to weight-related disorders.

It is vital to realize that these qualities generally interact and might vary greatly from person to person. Understanding why you are overweight is a complex process that includes personal thought, occasionally professional advice, and a commitment to achieving sustainable lifestyle changes. The journey towards healthier weight and overall well-being is quite personal, and acknowledging these contributing aspects is the first step towards significant transformation.

Understand Your Body's Signals:
Your body has a remarkable ability to transmit its requirements, often through subtle indicators that we have learned to disregard. This chapter is your guide to rediscovering and obeying these cues.

Hunger and Fullness: Your body's hunger and fullness signals are like an internal GPS that steers you toward a balanced diet. We're going to go into the necessity of reconnecting with these clues. You will learn to recognize the subtle grimace of hunger and the pleasant satisfaction of fullness. Knowing these signs, you can eat when you are genuinely hungry and stop when you are pleasantly full, developing a balanced relationship with the food.

Appetites: Appetites, normally seen negatively, can just be the way your body expresses its demands. We're going to investigate techniques to understand these instincts. Is it a yearning for something sweet, flavorful, or crunchy? Your body may be yearning for certain nutrients or simply for the pleasure of experiencing a preferred taste. We will offer techniques to satisfy desires correctly so that they do not lead to overindulgence.

Energy Levels: Your energy levels throughout the day convey essential information about your body's nutritional needs. We will study how to use your energy levels as a guide to when and what to eat. By aligning your meals with your body's energy needs, you can sustain continuous vigor, eliminating energy declines and cravings.

Break-Free Diet Culture:

This chapter is also a safe place to criticize the pervasive food culture that surrounds us. It is about releasing yourself from the relentless attack of external norms and laws, allowing you to listen and trust your own body.

Diet Misconceptions Debunked: We're going to uncover the reality behind the popular diet misconceptions that have fooled many about their health journeys. You will have a greater grasp of how these mistakes might impact your relationship with food. Armed with this information, you may make decisions that reflect the necessities of your body, not the expectations of society.

Refusing Food Guilt: Guilt typically accompanies our food decisions, throwing a shadow over our eating enjoyment. We will examine the damaging impact of food guilt and share methods to replace it with self-compassion and faith in your body's capacity to guide you. By removing the burden of guilt, you will be able to enjoy the pleasures of eating completely.

Honor Your Unique Body

There are no two similar bodies, and that's something to accept. In this chapter, you will discover how to honor your unique body and its requirements.

Body Diversity: We will celebrate the concept of body variety, highlighting that wellness is different for everyone. You will obtain an understanding of the beauty of diverse shapes and sizes of the body, knowing that there is no single route to well-being. It is about accepting and appreciating the natural form and size of your body while focusing on feeding it in a way that promotes real health and happiness.

Body Positivity: Embrace the positivity of the body, which is a crucial component of your path. We will share guidance on how to encourage self-love and acceptance, regardless of your size or body type. You will understand the power of positive speech and self-esteem as strategies to develop a more positive relationship with your body. By practicing self-compassion and appreciating the intrinsic value of your body, you will find a stronger feeling of confidence in yourself.

Practical Tools and Exercises:
Throughout this chapter, you will find practical activities and ways to help you reconnect with the knowledge of your body.

Cautious Eating Practices: You will explore cautious eating practices that urge you to slow down, savor each meal, and pay attention to your body's signs. These exercises can help you build a deeper connection with the food you consume and foster a more intuitive attitude toward eating.

Journaling Prompts: Journaling can be a fantastic tool for reflection and self-discovery. We will introduce you to diary questions that will motivate you to explore your relationship with food, your body, and your thoughts and feelings around food.

In Chapter 2, we encourage you to embark on a transformative journey of self-discovery, self-confidence, and self-compassion. It's about learning to trust your body's natural knowledge of nutrition, releasing yourself from the constraints of food culture, and celebrating the uniqueness of your body. At the end of this chapter, you will be equipped with the tools and information to make food choices that honor and support your well-being.

Trusting your body's knowledge is not just a key to lasting health but also a path to a fuller and more powerful existence. It is about creating a partnership with your body, built on confidence, respect, and self-compassion, that will guide you toward a future full of health, happiness, and harmony. So, let's dive together into this voyage of empowerment, where you will find that your body is truly a competent and trustworthy advisor when it comes to feeding.

Honor the Hunger and Satisfaction of your Body

In a world largely dominated by external food regulations and society's expectations to comply with specific dietary patterns, there is something blissfully liberating about evaluating the innate wisdom of your body when it comes to hunger and satiety. This practice, sometimes termed eating instinctively, is like rediscovering a forgotten art—a talent that can improve your connection with food and your general well-being.

Recognize Actual Hunger

Hunger is one of the most fundamental and honest messages from your body. It's a whisper from your body, reminding you it's time to eat. But in a culture that encourages us to repress our hunger or to conform to rigorous meal schedules, we may have been removed from this vital indicator.

Here's How to Reconnect with and Honor your Body's Hunger Signals

Listen Carefully: True hunger usually begins as a silent rumbling or a feeling of lightness in your stomach. It is not accompanied by specific impulses or urgency. Learn to notice these subtle signs and differentiate them from emotional or boring feeding.

Eat when you are Hungry: When you detect actual hunger, react to it. It's your body's technique for expressing its dietary needs. Delaying eating when you are hungry might lead to overfeeding later or a sensation of excessive deprivation, which can upset your connection with food.

Avoid Excessive Calorie Accounts: Concentrating too much on calorie counts or dish sizes can replace your natural hunger indices. Instead of tracking calories, focus on the quality of the food you choose and your body's signals of satiety.

Understanding Satiety

Just as it is crucial to observe your hunger marks, it is just as vital to know when your body communicates that it has had enough. It is the point of fullness or contentment, and it is your body's way of alerting you that it is satisfied with the food it has received.

Here's How to Honor the Indicators of Fullness of your Body

Eat Carefully: When you eat, be totally present. Be mindful of the aromas, tastes, and textures in your food. Eating intentionally helps you appreciate your food and become more aware of your body's indicators of satiety.

Monitor In During Meals: Take brief breaks during your meal to monitor your satiety. Put your fork on, take a few deep breaths, and ask yourself how content you are. Are you full or still hungry?

Avoid Excessive Food Intake: Overfeeding happens when you continue to eat past the point of satiety. This might lead to discomfort and guilt. By learning how to determine when you are no longer hungry, you may prevent overindulgence and maintain a balanced relationship with food.

The Benefits of Honoring Hunger and Satiety

Respecting your body's hunger and symptoms of satiety is not just about eating; it's about developing a profound connection between your mind and your body. This method offers a plethora of advantages:

Balanced Diet: When you eat in response to true hunger and stop when you are satisfied, you naturally gravitate towards balanced, healthful foods. Your body understands what it needs, and you grow better by picking nutrients that enhance your well-being.

Reduced Overindulgence: By paying attention to fullness indices, you prevent overeating, which can help with weight control and digestive comfort.

Improving the Relationship with Food: Respecting your body's cues promotes a pleasant relationship with food. You no longer regard food as something to manage or restrict but as a joyful and intuitive experience.

Emotional Wellbeing: Listening to your body's cues of hunger and satiety might boost your emotional well-being It eliminates the shame and anxiety associated with eating and fosters a sense of compassion and trust in your body.

The Voyage of Rediscovery

Honoring hunger and symptoms of satiety in your body is a journey of rediscovery, a trip that can take time and patience. This means not learning the teachings of food culture and recognizing yourself through the wisdom of your body.

As you embark on your quest, remember that it is entirely natural to make mistakes. You can sometimes eat when you are not hungry or quit before being satiated. It's part of the learning process. Each interaction offers an opportunity to improve your connection with your body and enhance your capacity to honor its messages.

Ultimately, this practice allows you to take charge of your eating choices, making them more intuitive and connected to your specific needs. It is about embracing the wisdom that dwells inside you and building a supportive relationship with your body that promotes your health, happiness, and well-being. So, let's begin on this adventure of tracking your body's hunger and signals of satiety together, unlocking the possibility for a more harmonious and satisfying interaction with food. Remember, your body is a trustworthy guide on the way to nutrition and well-being, and by listening to it, you can create a better and happier life.

Learn to Listen to Your Body's Needs

In our fast-paced environment, full of distractions and external influences, it is easy to lose contact with the intrinsic understanding of our body. Sometimes we find ourselves lost in the turmoil of life, ignoring the signs our bodies tell us. What if we could renew that connection? What if we could reclaim the art of listening to the needs of our body and using it as a compass for a better and happier life? Let us investigate this revolutionary journey of self-awareness and self-care even more deeply.

The Seal of Physical Sensations

Your body transmits its desires through a symphony of bodily sensations. These sensations are like whispers, lovely reminders that direct you to what your body requires.

Hunger Crazy: Stomach aches, lightness, or feeling empty are all indications of hunger. Learning to discern between actual physical hunger and emotional hunger is the first step to listening to your body. When you're hungry, it's the way your body signals that you need nourishment. Instead of dismissing it, accept it as a crucial indication to take care of yourself.

Thirst: Dehydration can occur as a dry mouth, headaches, or a general feeling of weariness. Paying attention to your body's symptoms of thirst is crucial to getting enough hydration. When you are thirsty, your body tells you it needs water. Ignoring this signal can lead to severe health hazards, so be careful to react fast.

Energy Levels: Your body's energy levels alter throughout the day. A feeling of tiredness may suggest that it is time to relax, while a burst of energy may mean that it's time for activity or action. Listening to these guidelines will help you enhance your everyday routines and perform according to your body's natural cycles.

Digestive Comfort: Physical discomfort after eating can be an indication that your body is not agreeing with a certain amount of food or portion. Listening to this advice could help you make better dietary choices and avoid things that may not agree with you. Your body offers essential information about what it needs for proper digestion and comfort.

Emotions as Messengers

Emotions, too, are part of this intricate communication system. They can be powerful messages from your body, informing you when something is amiss.

Stress: Experiencing stress or anxiety is the way your body informs you of potential threats. Learning to manage stress is a crucial component of self-care. When you experience stress, it is a signal that your body may need relaxation, deep breathing, or a respite from the source of stress.

Sadness: Sadness usually develops when you feel alienated or unhappy in a certain way. It's an invitation to evaluate what might be missing in your life. Instead of dismissing grief, honor it as an emotion that can lead you to greater self-awareness and constructive transformation.

Happiness: Joy and happiness are the ways your body appreciates moments of satisfaction and fulfillment. Recognizing and appreciating these emotions can contribute to general well-being. When you feel happiness, allow yourself to accept it and cherish it entirely. It's a reminder that your body responds positively to moments of joy.

Tuning into Full Consciousness:

Awareness is a strong skill that can help you listen to your body's desires. This means being totally present in the current moment and paying attention to your physical thoughts, emotions, and feelings without judgment.

Eat Carefully: Eating intentionally includes tasting every bite, chewing thoroughly, and paying attention to the flavors and textures of your meal. This activity can help you better detect the signals of hunger and satiety, as well as the enjoyment of eating.

Meditation: Meditation is a full-consciousness practice that helps you observe your physiological thoughts and sensations. It might help you become more conscious of the demands and feelings of your body. Regular practice of meditation can increase your ability to listen to your body and react with greater awareness.

Practice Self-Compassion:

Listening to your body's demands also entails practicing self-compassion. It means being fair to yourself, especially when you make choices that may not quite meet your body's requirements.

Forgiveness: If you eat too much or are not hungry, it is vital to forgive yourself. Self-criticism just creates tension, making it difficult to listen to your body in the future. Instead, regard these experiences as chances for growth and learning.

Feeding: Treat yourself with the same care and compassion that you would show to a good friend. Your body deserves your love and attention. Eating involves making decisions that prioritize your well-being, be it nutrition, exercise, or rest.

The Journey of Transformation:

Learning to listen to your body's needs is a transformative experience. It's about becoming the ally of your body rather than its opponent. It is a journey to self-discovery, self-care, and a greater connection with your physical and emotional well-being.

By recognizing the whispers of your body's feelings, emotions, and ideas, you may make decisions that meet your genuine requirements. This strategy helps you live a life that fosters health, happiness, and harmony.

So, let's walk into this adventure together, where you will learn to conform, listen, and respond to your body's requirements with care and knowledge. Your body is your loyal companion on this journey of life, and by nourishing this relationship, you can discover a healthier, happier, and more authentic version of yourself. Remember, your body is talking to you every day; all you have to do is listen. The more you practice this discipline, the more you will be in sync with the amazing symphony of sensations and emotions that guide you to a full and balanced life.

Building Trust and Intuition in Your Eating Habits

In a society overloaded with diet plans, food fads, and inconsistent nutrition advice, it's easy to feel overwhelmed and distant from our own bodies when it comes to eating. But there's a refreshing and deeply changing technique that can remodel your connection with food: building trust and intuition in your eating habits. This journey is about rekindling the innate wisdom inside you, empowering you to make food choices that truly nourish your body and spirit.

Understanding Trust and Intuition:

Building confidence and insight into your eating habits includes creating a strong, respectful collaboration with your body and its natural signs. It's a departure from severe norms and external guidelines and an embrace of self-compassion and self-awareness.

Listening to Your Body:

Hunger Signs: Trusting your body's indications of hunger is vital. Your body detects when it needs nutrition. Rather than ignoring or suppressing hunger, honor it as a biological cue that demands attention. Listening to your body's hunger cues helps you consume when you actually need nourishment, supporting balanced nutrition. Pay attention to the tiny indicators of hunger, from the quiet rumbling of your stomach to the slight fall in energy levels. These cues are your body's approach to notifying you it's time to eat.

Fullness Signs: Intuition in eating also entails identifying your body's indications of fullness. It's about stopping when your content is not full. This exercise minimizes overeating and builds a positive connection with food. Your body delivers cues of fullness, such as a feeling of contentment and a steady decrease in hunger. Learning to comprehend and heed these indicators helps you create a natural sense of portion management.

Embracing Mindfulness

Mindfulness is a wonderful technique for cultivating trust and intuition in your eating habits. It requires being entirely present throughout meals, relishing each bite, and paying attention to the sensations and flavors of your food.

Sensory Experience: Engage your senses when you eat. Notice the textures, colors, and scents of your meal. This concentration allows you to actually savor your food and be in harmony with your body's responses. It helps you savor each bite and improves your awareness of how different foods make you feel.

Chew Slowly: Eating slowly and digesting your meal completely not only improves digestion but also offers you time to observe your body's fullness indicators. It's a simple yet powerful way to increase your food intuition. Chewing slowly also allows you to properly savor the taste and texture of your food.

Breaking Free from Diet Culture:

Building confidence and intuition in your eating habits frequently requires defying the dominant diet culture that surrounds us.

Diet Fallacies: recognize and reject classic diet fallacies that promote external control over your eating habits. Embrace the notion that your body has its own wisdom and that there is no one-size-fits-all approach to food. Understand that what works for one person may not work for another, and that's totally alright.

Reject Food Guilt: Diet culture sometimes comes with a side plate of food guilt. It's vital to reject this guilt and replace it with self-compassion. Trust that your body can guide you to make balanced judgments without the weight of shame. If you periodically indulge in a treat or eat for comfort, see it as a normal part of your relationship with food, not as a failure.

The Role of Intuition:

Intuition is a valuable friend in your journey. It's that gut feeling or inner understanding that helps you make choices associated with your body's demands.

Food Choice Intuition: As you practice listening to your body, you'll notice your intuition guiding you towards foods that make you feel good and energized. Trust these desires, as they often lead to healthy decisions. You might find yourself reflexively leaning towards fruits and vegetables when your body demands vitamins and minerals, or lean proteins when it requires fuel.

Emotional Eating: Your sense of smell also enables your body to differentiate between hunger and sensitive meals. When you find yourself reaching for food in response to emotions, pause and ask yourself if your body is genuinely hungry or seeking comfort in other ways. This self-awareness helps you handle emotional demands without turning to food as a key coping mechanism.

The Transformational Journey:

Building confidence and intuition in your eating habits is a transformative experience. It's a transformation from external control to inner awareness, from guilt to self-compassion, and from confusion to clarity.

By accepting hunger and fullness cues, practicing mindfulness, and rejecting the constraints of diet culture, you'll go on a journey that nourishes not only your body but also your soul. This journey is about building a fundamental connection with your body's natural intelligence, knowing he holds the secret to your well-being.

So, let's journey together into this empowerment adventure, where you will learn to trust your body's messages, nurture intuition in your eating habits, and build a relationship with food that is built on self-compassion and authenticity. By doing this, you will discover the transformational potential of nourishing your body and soul, leading to a life full of health, happiness, and harmony. Trust yourself; you have all the wisdom you need within yourself. Your body is not merely a conduit for food; it is a profound source of guidance and intuition, ready to guide you toward a more balanced and fulfilling life

Chapter 3: Eating Carefully for Weight Loss

In a world where rapid diets and weight loss trends are continually capturing our attention, the concept of mindful eating is a novel and sustainable method of obtaining a healthy weight. In this chapter, we'll explore the discipline of conscious eating, a practice that goes beyond the constraints of conventional diets and helps you generate fundamental and lasting changes in your relationship with food and your body.

What Works for Overweight People:

Constant Effort: Consistency is the heart of successful weight management for people who are overweight. It is vital to recognize that sustained transformation takes time. Instead of anticipating abrupt transformations, individuals should focus on modesty and continual improvement. Simple, minor modifications in eating habits and exercise routines can produce huge long-term consequences.

Set Realistic Objectives: Setting achieved goals is an important aspect of effective weight management. Rather than focusing on enormous and inaccessible aspirations, it is more useful to develop feasible and smaller stages. These milestones offer a sense of achievement and training, propelling individuals toward their ultimate goals. Celebrating these accomplishments along the path helps increase confidence and drive.

Meal Planning: Meal planning is a realistic strategy that can substantially benefit those who are overweight. By preparing meals in advance, individuals can make intentional, health-conscious decisions. This strategy helps to select nutritious, well-balanced foods and lowers the possibility of impulsive, less healthy dietary decisions. In addition, meal planning aids with quantity control, which is vital for calorie management.

Hydration: Adequate hydration is often undervalued yet plays a crucial role in weight management. Staying sufficiently hydrated benefits overall health and can help regulate hunger. Sometimes, thirst is confused with hunger, leading individuals to consume unnecessary calories. Drinking a proper amount of water throughout the day will help to minimize this false hunger signal and aid in healthier weight management.

What Does Not wWork for Overweight People?

Skip meals: Skipping meals, especially breakfast, is not an appropriate method for people who are trying to manage their weight. This behavior might lead to an increase in hunger later in the day, which usually ends in overeating or a less nutritional meal choice. Regular meals, especially those with balanced nutrients, support metabolism and help maintain stable blood sugar levels.

Excessive Concentration on the Scale: Placing too much emphasis on the number represented on the scale can be damaging. Weight changes normally due to variables, including water retention and muscle growth. Relying entirely on the amount of progress can lead to frustration and disappointment, especially if the focus is on short-term fluctuations rather than long-term trends.

Compared With Others: Comparing one weight loss vacation to others can be depressing. Each individual's physiology and circumstances are unique, resulting in varied rates of improvement. It is vital to focus on personal goals and achievements rather than drawing external comparisons. Personal achievements and improvement are the fundamental metrics of success.

Ignorance of Emotional Well-being: Emotional well-being is an important aspect of effective weight management. Neglected stress, anxiety, and self-health can jeopardize even the finest weight loss attempts. Addressing emotional components through mindfulness activities, relaxation techniques or counseling is vital to sustainable success.

Elimination of Whole Food Groups: Extreme diets that completely exclude important food groups, such as carbs or lipids, are frequently unsustainable and potentially harmful. These diets can lead to nutritional imbalances and make it difficult to maintain a balanced and varied diet. A balanced plan that includes a wide variety of nutrients is vital for long-term success.

Ignore Indicators of Satiety: Over-eating, or eating beyond the fullness point, is a regular problem that might compromise the effectiveness of weight loss.

Adjusting bodily indicators for hunger and satiety is crucial. Learning to notice these indicators and respond accordingly helps individuals manage their nutritional intake more successfully and maintain a healthy weight.

Understanding these extra realities of what works and what doesn't work for persons who are overweight provides a holistic view of effective weight management techniques. It emphasizes the necessity of sustainable and balanced techniques that prioritize physical and mental well-being throughout the road toward obtaining a dining a healthier weight.

The Essence of Careful Feeding:

At its foundation, eating wisely aims to foster a higher awareness of your eating experience. It is an invitation to bring the full consciousness, or the awareness of the present moment, to your meals. This practice inspires you to:

Taste every Bite: Instead of hurrying through your meals, take the time to taste each piece. Pay close attention to the flavor, purpose, and smell of your food. This not only boosts your meal pleasure but also allows you to grow more comfortable with your body's signals of hunger and satiety. When you like your food, you naturally slow down, which makes it simpler to recognize when you are satisfied. This can avoid overfeeding.

Eat with Intention: Eating carefully urges you to eat consciously, matching your choices with your body's demands. It entails picking foods that nourish and make you feel well. It's about going from careless and impulsive eating to making careful selections about what you eat and when. When you eat consciously, you are less likely to absorb meals that do not encourage your well-being, which can assist in reducing weight and overall health.

Honor Your Body: Eating wisely teaches you to honor your body's appetite and indicators of satiety. You eat when you are hungry and you stop when you're satisfied, not when other factors demand it. This strategy naturally aids weight management by preventing overfeeding and underfeeding. By obeying the cues of your body, you build a more intuitive and balanced relationship with food.

Cultivate Consciousness: It is also about growing awareness of the triggers and emotional eating routines. By recognizing when and why you eat for emotional reasons, you acquire the ability to address the underlying feelings in a more effective way. Eating emotionally can often contribute to weight gain, therefore becoming more conscious of these behaviors is vital for weight management.

Eat Cautiously and Lose Weight:

While eating properly is not a rapid reaction to weight loss, it offers a permanent approach to obtaining a healthy weight. Here's how:

Reduces Overeating: By paying attention to your body's cues of satiety, you're less likely to overeat. This can lead to a slow and consistent decrease in calorie consumption, assisting with weight loss or maintenance. A smart diet helps you avoid the frequent pitfalls of irresponsible nibbling and huge meals.

Balanced Choice: Eating attentively naturally supports balanced meal choices. As you get more accustomed to your body's requirements, you're probably picking healthy foods that supply important nutrients without additional calories. You may discover that you naturally gravitate towards fruits, vegetables, lean meats, and whole grains, which aid with weight loss.

Emotional Eating Awareness: A mindful diet will help you identify sensitive eating patterns that are frequently linked to weight gain. By managing emotional triggers in a healthier way, you lessen the need for food as a management tool. This knowledge helps you make decisions that match your body's hunger rather than your emotional desires.

Long-term Sustainability: Unlike restrictive diets that typically lead to weight recovery, mindful eating is a sustainable discipline. It is a diet regimen that can begin throughout your life, promoting sustained weight management. Instead of looking at it as a short-term treatment, consider it a lasting commitment to your well-being.

Practical Advice for a Cautious Diet:
To start eating properly for weight loss, consider these practical tips:

Slow Down: Eat at a relaxed pace, taking the time to chew each item fully. This permits your body to feel full more effectively and reduces the habit of eating on autopilot.

Portion Control: Use smaller plates and utensils to encourage portion management. This helps to avoid overeating by visually fooling your brain into thinking that you are eating more. Be aware of portion size and avoid the desire to come back for seconds without verifying your hunger signs.

Eliminate Distractions: Eat without distractions such as TV or smartphones. Concentrate entirely on the act of eating and the sensory sensation of your food. This practice raises your awareness of the flavors and sensations of your food.

Check-in with Hunger: Before eating, take the time to check your hunger levels. Are you genuinely hungry, or do you eat by habit or emotion? This break helps you make careful choices about how to eat and how much to ingest.

Exercise of Appreciation: Express your thankfulness for your food. Recognize the labor that has gone into growth, preparation, and service. This can boost your enjoyment of your meals and establish a nice relationship with the food.

The Mind-body Connection:

Eating mindfully isn't just about what you put on your plate; it's about developing a healthy mind-body relationship. By practicing full mindfulness at meals, you establish a foundation of self-knowledge and compassion that extends beyond food and influences other elements of your life.

As you continue on your path to eating carefully for weight loss, realize that this is not a goal but a lifelong habit. It is about enjoying the present moment, creating a harmonious connection with food and, ultimately, achieving a healthy weight while savoring each meal's richness. So, let's go on this innovative journey together, where you'll discover the full potential of mindful eating as a lasting and pleasurable weight management technique. By integrating full awareness into your eating habits, you will not only support your weight objectives but also increase your general well-being, a thoughtful tongue at a time.

Explore the Concept of Conscious Food

In a culture that often favors speed, convenience, and multitasking, the idea of mindful eating provides a refreshing alternative. It is a manner of nourishing your body that transcends the act of eating and becomes a deep practice of self-awareness, self-care, and appreciation for the simple but crucial activity of ingesting food.

What is Conscious Eating?

At its core, eating thoughtfully is the practice of applying consciousness, or knowledge of the present moment, to your meals and snacks. It's about activating all your senses - sight, smell, taste, touch, and even sound - when you eat. This practice inspires you to:

Slow Down: Instead of racing through meals, eating attentively forces you to slow down and savor each bite. Pay attention to your taste and smell. This not only boosts your meal pleasure but also allows you to grow more comfortable with your body's signals of hunger and satiety. When you like your food, you naturally slow down, which makes it simpler to recognize when you are satisfied. This can avoid overfeeding.

Attention: Attentive diet urges you to pay full attention to your food and the act of eating. It implies eating without distractions such as watching TV, smartphones, or work. When you focus totally on your food, you become more attentive to the hunger and satiety signals from your body.

Watch Your Body: It asks you to pay attention to the symptoms of hunger and satiety in your body. You eat when you are hungry and you stop when you're satisfied, instead of finishing what's on your plate or eating on external schedules.

Watch Emotional Feeding: Eating carefully also involves observing emotional eating tendencies. It helps you recognize when you eat in response to emotions, such as tension, boredom, or depression. This information helps you respond to emotional demands in a more constructive way.

Benefits of Eating Carefully:

The practice of mindful eating provides a wide range of benefits that go beyond weight management alone:

Weight Control: A healthy diet can help reduce weight by avoiding overeating and increasing portion control. When you pay attention to your body's cues of hunger and satiety, you're less likely to eat excess calories.

Improving Digestion: Bite food deeply and consume attentively to help digest. It allows your body to break down meals more efficiently and absorb nutrients more effectively.

More Enjoyment: Eating carefully often leads to more enjoyment with your meals. By taking each bite and fully tasting the flavors, you might find greater pleasure in your food.

Emotional Wellbeing: This practice can also enhance emotional well-being. It helps you build a healthy relationship with food and a deeper knowledge of how emotions affect your eating patterns.

Reduces Stress: Eating sensibly can lessen food-related stress. It eliminates the strain of following tight diets and offers a more relaxed and pleasurable dining experience.

How to Practice a Careful Diet:

If you are new to eating mindfully, here are some practical methods to get started.

Choose a Peaceful Environment: Find a quiet and comfortable area to dine without distractions. Turn off the TV, put your phone down, and establish a peaceful atmosphere.

Engage your Senses: Before taking your first bite, take time to savor your cuisine with your senses. Watch the colors, textures, and scents of your food. This sensory awareness can strengthen your interaction with your meal.

Chew Gently: while you eat, chew each item slowly and carefully. Pay attention to the taste, texture and smell of your food.

Between the bites, put your utensils or food and take a pause. This little break helps you check with your body and examine your hunger level.

Eat Deliberately: Keep eating deliberately, keeping present with each bite. Be conscious of the feelings of fullness as they emerge.

Watch Emotions: If you identify emotional triggers for eating, recognize them without judgment. Ask yourself if you are actually hungry or if there is an emotional need that you may meet differently.

Express Thankfulness: After your meal, take time to express your gratitude for the food you have received. This exercise helps to create a good relationship with the food.

The Transformational Path of Conscious Food:
Exploring the concept of mindful eating isn't just about changing the way you eat; it's a transforming journey of self-discovery and self-care. It is an opportunity to cultivate a deeper connection with your body and develop a more harmonious relationship with food.

When you embark on this route, remember that eating properly is not a matter of perfection, but of activity. It is about creating a thoughtful attitude to the food that you can keep with you throughout your life, improve your general well-being, and help you make choices that match your body's requirements. So let's explore this interesting adventure together, where you will find the delight of sustaining your body and mind with an attentive consciousness, one food at a time. By integrating full awareness into your eating habits, you will not only support your weight goals but also improve your general quality of life, one moment at a time.

Cultivate Awareness During Meals

In the frequentization of modern life, meals are often stuck between homework, consigned to the background while we work, watch TV, or surf on our smartphones. The concept of greater awareness during meals allows us to get out of this frenetic pattern and change our eating experience into an attentive and nutritious exercise.

Why Cultivate Attentiveness throughout Meals?

When we eat mindlessly, we lack the richness of the food we swallow, and we distance ourselves from the signals from our bodies. Cultivating awareness during meals has a number of benefits that can boost our physical and emotional well-being:

Pleasure Enhancement: When you eat thoughtfully, you savor every bite. You love the textures, aromas, and fragrances of your food, transforming each meal into a sensuous experience. Whether it's the crispiness of a fresh salad, the heat of a bowl of soup, or the sweetness of a piece of ripe fruit, awareness boosts the pleasure you obtain from eating.

Improving Digestion: Eating your food fully and eating slowly helps with better digestion. It allows your body to break down meals more efficiently and absorb nutrients efficiently. When you eat intentionally, you are less likely to lose food, which could result in digestive pain. Instead, you allow your digestive system to function efficiently.

Recognize Hunger and Fullness: Being mindful throughout meals helps you reconnect with your body's cues of hunger and satiety. This implies that you are more likely to eat when you actually are hungry and quit when you are satisfied, which improves weight management. It is an excellent method against overeating and mindless consumption of excess calories.

Stress Reduction: Eating with reflection helps alleviate the tension and anxiety linked with food. It fosters a feeling of calm and relaxation during meals, decreasing the rush and turmoil that generally accompanies eating in a hurry. Instead of treating meals as another item on your to-do list, it becomes a period of quiet and food.

Emotional Balance: By paying attention to your eating habits, you become more aware of the emotional triggers for overeating or poor choices. This understanding permits you to manage emotional demands in healthier ways. Instead of turning to food as a way to cope with stress, sadness, or boredom, you can build alternate tactics for mental well-being.

Practical Techniques to Cultivate Alertness During Meals:

To include this practice into your everyday routine, consider the following tips:

Create a Tanquil Environment: Find a quiet area for dinner, free of distractions like TV or your phone. Create a nice setting that encourages relaxing. If feasible, dine in a place with natural light or peaceful decor to improve the ambiance.

Start with Thankfulness: Take a moment to express your gratitude for your meal. Think about the labor that has been done to grow, prepare, and serve the food. This simple action can shift your outlook and build a positive relationship with what you are going to eat. Gratitude adds a layer of awareness to your meal, reminding you to appreciate the availability of food.

Engage your Senses: Before taking your first bite, observe your meal with all your senses. Note the colors, textures, and smells of the meal. This sensory connection ties you to the present moment and boosts your appreciation of the meal. The vibrant colors of a salad, the earthly perfume of a heated soup bowl, and the relaxing heat of a freshly brewed cup of tea can all be sources of sensory pleasure.

Chew Slowly and Carefully: while you eat, chew each piece gently and thoroughly. This not only assists digestion but also allows you to completely experience the flavors and feelings of your food. It's a way to recognize the work that served cooking your dinner. Each item becomes an opportunity to taste and appreciate the gourmet beauty before you.

Between the bites, put your utensils or food and take a pause. Take the time to check your physique. Are you still hungry or are you starting to feel full? This strategy helps you listen to your body's instructions. It's a reminder to eat in reaction to your body's demands rather than external messages.

Be Present: Keep your attention on the food in front of you. Avoid hurrying to eat or letting your attention pass. If your mind starts to drift, gradually turn your attention to the process of eating. It is an exercise of full consciousness, to root yourself in the present moment.

Enjoy Silence: Embrace silence during meals. Instead of filling the air with discussion or diversions, embrace calm. This silence can be a crucial component of your mindful eating experience. It allows you to totally immerse yourself in the act of eating, free from outside discussion or noise.

The Transformative Power of Cultivating Consciousness:

Cultivating mindfulness during meals is more than just changing the way you eat, it's a transformative practice that may strengthen your general connection with food and your body. It asks you to slow down, enjoy the present, and reconnect with the fundamental task of nourishing yourself.

When you integrate this practice into your regular life, remember that it is not about perfection, but development. Small efforts towards increased awareness during meals can lead to substantial changes in the way you eat and how you interact with food. By growing awareness at the dinner table, you travel a journey of self-discovery, improved digestion, and a more balanced and harmonic approach to eating. So, let's build mindfulness during the meals together, and by doing so, let's find the huge potential of each mouthful to nourish not only your body but also your mind. By integrating full awareness into your eating habits, you will not only support your weight goals but also improve your general quality of life, one moment at a time.

Use Conscious Diet as a Technique for Lasting Weight Loss

In a world often focused on fast solutions and modest diets, the idea of choosing a cautious diet as a sustainable weight loss technique looks like a fresh and revolutionary method. It's a journey that goes beyond typical diet techniques, allowing you to go on a path of self-discovery, self-care, and sustainable change in your relationship with food and your body.

The Essence of Careful Diet for Weight Loss:

At its foundation, eating wisely aims to foster a higher awareness of your eating experience. It is an invitation to apply the entire consciousness, or the awareness of the present moment, to your meals and snacks. This practice inspires you to:

Taste every Bite: Instead of hurrying through your meals, take the time to taste each piece. Pay attention to your taste and smell. This not only boosts your meal pleasure but also allows you to grow more comfortable with your body's signals of hunger and satiety. When you like your food, you naturally slow down, which makes it simpler to recognize when you are satisfied. This can avoid overfeeding.

Eat with Intention: Eating carefully urges you to eat consciously, matching your choices with your body's demands. It involves choosing foods that nourish and make you feel good. It's about moving from careless and impulsive eating to making careful decisions about what you eat and when you consume.

When you eat consciously, you are less likely to absorb meals that do not encourage your well-being, which can assist in reducing weight and overall health.

Honor your Body: Eating wisely teaches you to honor your body's appetite and indicators of satiety. You eat when you are hungry and you stop when you're satisfied, not when other factors demand it. This strategy naturally aids weight management by preventing overfeeding and underfeeding. By obeying the cues of your body, you build a more intuitive and balanced relationship with food.

Cultivate Consciousness: It is also about growing awareness of the triggers and emotional eating routines. By recognizing when and why you eat for emotional reasons, you acquire the ability to address the underlying feelings in a more effective way. Eating emotionally can often contribute to weight gain, therefore becoming more conscious of these behaviors is vital for weight management.

Eat Cautiously and Lose Weight:

While eating properly is not a rapid reaction to weight loss, it offers a permanent approach to obtaining and dining a healthy weight. Here's how:

Reduces Overeating: By paying attention to your body's cues of satiety, you're less likely to overeat. This can lead to a slow and consistent decrease in calorie consumption, assisting with weight loss or maintenance. A smart diet helps you avoid the frequent pitfalls of irresponsible nibbling and huge meals.

Balanced Choice: Eating attentively naturally supports balanced meal choices. As you get more accustomed to your body's requirements, you're probably picking healthy foods that supply important nutrients without additional calories. You may discover that you naturally gravitate towards fruits, vegetables, lean meats, and whole grains, which aid with weight loss.

Emotional eating helps you discover the emotional eating habits commonly associated with weight gain. By managing emotional triggers in a healthier way, you lessen the need for food as a management tool. This knowledge helps you make decisions that match your body's hunger rather than your emotional desires.

Long-term sustainability: Unlike restrictive diets that typically lead to weight recovery, mindful eating is a sustainable discipline. It is a diet regimen that can beined throughout your life, promoting sustained weight management. Instead of looking at it as a short-term treatment, consider it a lasting commitment to your well-being.

Practical Ideas for Utilizing a Cautious Diet for Weight Loss:

To effectively employ mindful eating as a sustained weight loss approach, consider these practical tips:

Slow Down: Eat at a relaxed pace, taking the time to chew each item fully. This permits your body to feel full more effectively and reduces the habit of eating on autopilot.

Portion Control: Use smaller plates and utensils to encourage portion management. This helps to avoid overeating by visually fooling your brain into thinking that you are eating more. Be aware of portion size and avoid the desire to come back for seconds without verifying your hunger signs.

Eliminate Distractions: Eat without distractions such as TV or smartphones. Concentrate entirely on the act of eating and the sensory sensation of your food. This practice raises your awareness of the flavors and sensations of your food.

Check-in with Hunger: Before eating, take the time to check your hunger levels. Are you genuinely hungry, or do you eat by habit or emotion? This break helps you make careful choices about how to eat and how much to ingest.

Exercise of Appreciation: Express your thankfulness for your food. Recognize the labor that has gone into growth, preparation, and service. This can boost your enjoyment of your meals and establish a nice relationship with the food.

The Mind-body Connection:

Eating mindfully isn't just about what you put on your plate; it's about developing a healthy mind-body relationship. By practicing full mindfulness at meals, you establish a foundation of self-knowledge and compassion that extends beyond food and influences other elements of your life.

Embrace a Lifelong Journey:

As you continue on your journey to employ cautious eating for lasting weight loss, realize that this is not a destination but a lifelong habit. It is about enjoying the present moment, creating a harmonious connection with food, and, ultimately, achieving a healthy weight while savoring each meal's richness. By integrating full awareness into your eating habits, you will not only support your weight objectives but also increase your general well-being, a thoughtful tongue at a time. This practice is not only a tool for weight loss but also a doorway to a more balanced and fulfilled life.

Chapter 4: Adoption of Food Freedom

In a world typically characterized by severe dietary laws, calorie tracking, and dietary limitations, the concept of choosing food freedom looks like a liberating and reinforcing way to have a healthier and happier relationship with food. This chapter urges you to liberate yourself from the chains of food culture and find the true meaning of balance and autonomy when it comes to your eating habits.

Adopt Food Freedom

A Lifestyle Diet for Weight Loss:

Balanced Nutrition: Adopt a balanced and diversified diet that incorporates a wide range of nutrients. Prioritize entire foods such as fruit, vegetables, lean protein, whole grains, and healthy fats. These meals provide critical nutrients, fiber, and sustained energy, helping you feel satiated while limiting calorie consumption.

Portion Control: Practice portion control while keeping portion measurements in mind. Use smaller plates to prevent overflowing your plate, and heed your body's appetite and indicators of satiety. Avoid eating directly from the package, as this might lead to mindless munching.

frequent Meals: Establish a routine of eating frequent, balanced meals throughout the day. Skipping meals can lead to overeating later owing to increased hunger. Include nutritious proteins, fiber, and fats in each meal to maintain stable blood sugar levels.

Eat Carefully: Adopt careful eating habits. Pay attention to the sensory experience of eating, and tasting the flavors, textures, and fragrances of your food. Eat without distractions, such as screens or work, to participate completely in your meals.

Hydration: Stay well hydrated by drinking water throughout the day. Sometimes thirst is confused with hunger, resulting in unnecessary calorie consumption. Drinking water can help regulate appetite and enhance overall health.

Habits for Continual Weight Loss:

Regular Physical Activity: Incorporate regular physical activity into your regimen. Target a combination of cardiovascular workouts, strength training, and flexibility. Find activities you like to make fitness a lifelong habit.

Meal Planning: Plan your meals and snacks in advance. This technique helps you make healthier choices and minimizes the possibility of impulsive, less nutritious choices. It also helps with portion management and prevents food waste.

Journaling: Keep a food record to chronicle your eating patterns and feelings linked to eating. This self-awareness can assist in identifying emotional or mindless feeding behaviors and guide your decisions.

Support System: seek help from a dietician, therapist, or a recognized weight loss group. Having a support system provides guidance, encouragement, and responsibility for your weight reduction journey.

Self-Compassion: Practice self-compassion and avoid being overly critical of yourself. Understand that chess is a natural part of the trip. Instead of perceiving them as failures, see them as chances for learning and progress.

Management Skills: Develop healthy stress management skills and emotional challenges that do not involve overeating. Explore relaxation, meditation, or leisure practices that provide emotional release without turning to food.

Social and Environmental Awareness: Be conscious of your social and environmental influences. Surround yourself with friends and family who support you and encourage your healthy choices. Create an environment at home and at work that fosters healthy choices.

Focus on Consistency rather than Perfection: Sustainable weight loss means making slow and continuous adjustments over time. Avoid severe diets or quick weight-loss regimens that are difficult to sustain.

Long-term View: Keep a long-term view. Weight management is a lifelong journey, not a quick solution. Adopt the premise that your lifestyle and eating habits are for sustainable health and well-being.

By adopting this balanced eating lifestyle and incorporating these behaviors into your daily routine, you can encourage steady and permanent weight loss while emphasizing your entire health and well-being. Remember that patience, self-compassion, and a long-term perspective are key to sustainable success.

The Essence of Food Freedom:

At its foundation, the adoption of food independence aims to establish a sense of autonomy and confidence in your own body. It is an attitude towards food that realizes that food is not just food; it is a source of joy, culture, and connection. Food

Freedom encourages you to:

Skip the Restriction: Instead of following tight diets or labeling foods as "good" or "bad," food freedom asks you to let go of dietary restraints. It's about accepting the idea that all foods serve a function in your diet, and no food should be out of line.

Tune in your Body: Food freedom requires you to listen to your body's instincts, understanding that it knows what it needs. This means eating when you are hungry and giving up when you're satisfied, rather than following external norms or schedules.

Cultivate a Positive Relationship with Food: This strategy entails building a good and caring relationship with food. It encourages you to enjoy your meals without guilt, savoring the sensations and experiences that food brings.

Eat carefully. Adoption of food independence usually goes hand in hand with a careful diet. It's about appreciating the present moment during meals, eating purposefully, and paying attention to your body's signs.

The Benefits of Food Freedom:

Adopting food independence has various benefits that can improve your connection with food and your general well-being.

Reduces Stress: Removing dietary limitations and the need to follow restrictive diets can greatly lessen the tension associated with eating. It eliminates the tension and worry associated with "cheating days" or the breaking of dietary norms.

Increased Pleasure: Food freedom allows you to fully appreciate the pleasure of eating. You can enjoy the tastes and textures of your favorite dishes without feeling awful. This enjoyment can lead to a more fulfilling and sustainable way of eating.

Improved Body Image: By taking a more tolerant and empathetic approach to your body and its demands, you can enjoy benefits in body image and self-esteem. Food freedom asks you to appreciate your body for what it can do rather than condemn it for what you eat.

Eat Intuitively: Embrace food freedom, which often corresponds to an intuitive diet, a practice that encourages you to follow your body's cues of hunger and satiety. This can support good weight management and lower the danger of overeating.

Long-term Sustainability: Unlike restrictive diets that are difficult to maintain over time, food freedom is a sustainable approach to food. It is a way of sustaining yourself that may be done throughout your life, assuring long-term health and well-being.

Practical Recommendations for Adopting Food Freedom:

Let Food Labels Pass: Release the idea of classifying foods as "good" or "bad". All foods have their place in a balanced diet, and no item should be condemned or celebrated.

Listen to your Body: Download the signals of hunger and satiety in your body. You eat when you're hungry and you stop when you're full. Trust your body to comprehend what it needs.

Ditch Dieting Jargon: Avoid employing diet jargon or participating in negative self-talk about food or your physique. Replace words like "deceive" or "guilt" with more positive and attentive language.

Eat Carefully: Incorporate careful eating into your meals. Slow down, chew every bite, and savor the sensory sensation of food. Look at how the different foods make you feel, pay attention.

Cultivate Self-compassion: Be kind to yourself. Understand that you're eating habits may not be flawless, and it's acceptable. Treat yourself with the same care and forgiveness you would give a friend.

The Freedom to Prosper Health

Adopting food freedom is not just about what you eat; it is about the Freedom to thrive in every aspect of your life. It is a road of self-discovery, self-acceptance, and self-care. By renouncing restrictive diets and adopting a balanced and intuitive approach to diet, you can find greater peace, joy, and fulfillment in your connection with food and your body.

When you enter this chapter, remember that food freedom is not a destination but a lifelong exploration. It's a process of learning, growing, and expanding in your connection with the interview. By incorporating the principles of food independence into your life, you support not only your physical health but also your emotional well-being and create a deeper awareness of the richness of life's flavors. So let's go along this path of adopting food freedom together, unlocking the real potential of food as a source of nutrition, joy, and empowerment. By doing this, you will learn that true freedom is to embrace and enjoy the incredible tapestry of foods that make life both tasty and meaningful.

Incorporate Physical Activity into Your Schedule

In our quest for a better and more balanced existence, it is crucial to realize the enormous impact of physical activity on our overall well-being. Beyond the areas of diet and nutrition, regular exercise is an essential component that can boost our health, help sustain weight management, and contribute to a better and fuller life. In this chapter, we will explore the relevance of physical activity in your daily routine and learn how it can be a source of joy, empowerment, and sustainable transformation.

The Power of Physical Activity:

Physical activity is not only a way to burn calories; it is a celebration of what your body is capable of achieving. Here is why including regular physical activity in your routine is crucial:

Improved Metabolism: Engaging in activity cranks up your metabolic rate, making your body more efficient in burning calories. This increase in metabolism can help weight management by helping you burn calories, even when you are resting.

Mood Enhancement: Exercise is a natural mood booster. It triggers the release of endorphins, the "feel good" hormones that reduce stress, alleviate anxiety and fight depression. Regular physical activity can be a potent cure for the strains of ordinary life.

Increased Energy: Paradoxically, participating in physical activity provides an explosion of energy. Regular exercise can minimize feelings of exhaustion and boost your overall energy, allowing you to handle daily responsibilities with more enthusiasm.

Improving Cardiovascular Health: Cardiovascular exercises such as walking, running, and swimming strengthen your heart and improve your circulatory system. This not only minimizes the risk of heart disease but also promotes your overall cardiovascular health.

Better Sleep: Multiple physical activity promotes a good sleep patterns. It can help you fall asleep faster, enjoy deeper sleep cycles, and wake up feeling more refreshed and renewed.

Stronger Muscles and Bones: Weight-loaded workouts, such as resistance training, increase muscle strength and bone density. This is important as we age, as it can help prevent diseases such as osteoporosis and maintain overall physical function.

Improved Cognitive Function: Physical activity is not only healthy for your body; it is fantastic for your brain as well. Exercise was linked to better memory, greater cognitive function, and higher concentration.

Incorporate Physical Activity into Your Daily Life:

The thought of introducing regular physical activity into your daily routine should not be intimidating or long. Here are some practical tips to make it a natural and pleasurable part of your life:

Find the Hobbies you Like

The answer to maintaining fitness is to select fit-ups that actually bring you pleasure. Whether it's dancing, hiking, cycling, practicing yoga, or simply enjoying quiet walks in nature, discover activities that correspond with your interests and inclinations.

Start Slowly: If you are new to exercising or back after a break, start carefully and gradually adding intensity and length. It is crucial to listen to your body and prevent excessive exertion, which makes the practice more practical and pleasurable.

Set Realistic Goals: Set feasible goals depending on your current fitness level and schedule. These goals bring inspiration and a sense of accomplishment as you improve in your fitness journey.

Incorporate Variety: Variety not only makes your workout regimen interesting but also guarantees that you engage different muscle groups. Consider a blend of aerobic workouts (such as rapid walking or jogging), strength training (with weights or resistance bands), and flexibility exercising (like yoga or stretching routines).

Make it Social: Exercise with friends, and family, or attending a group class can make physical activity more pleasant and provide a social element that adds motivation and responsibility.

Prioritize Coherence: Cohesion is vital to achieving the advantages of physical activity. Target for regular, shorter, rather than occasional, long workouts. Even short and frequent episodes of activity can be advantageous.

Plan: Treat exercise like you would any other visit. Plan your training sessions in your daily or weekly agenda, ensuring that they become non-negotiable commitments.

Stay Hydrated: good hydration is crucial for good training. Drink water before, during, and after your workouts to maintain optimal performance and recuperation.

Listen to your Body: Pay attention to your body's footprints throughout physical exercise. If you encounter pain, discomfort, or extreme weariness, it is entirely reasonable to take a break, adjust your workout, or seek support from a fitness specialist.

Recognize Progress: recognize your fitness achievements, no matter how modest they may appear. Recognize advances in your stamina, strength, flexibility, and overall well-being. These milestones could act as motivating markers in your journey for fitness.

Make It a Lifestyle:

Incorporating physical activity into your routine goes beyond reaching a specific body weight or form; it is about adopting a lifestyle that values movement, vitality, and holistic well-being. It is a journey of self-care and self-discovery that celebrates the vast potential of your body, regardless of age or fitness level.

So, while you explore the pages of this chapter, remember that physical activity is not a duty but a chance for growth and pleasure. By weaving action into your everyday life, you not only support your weight management goals but also start a journey of empowerment and comprehensive well-being. The beauty of physical activity resides in its ability to enrich every element of your life, from physical health to mental and emotional well-being. Rally these sneakers, stretch those muscles, and dance at the rhythm of a vigorous and exciting existence.

Understand the Value of Self-Care

In the darkness of our everyday lives, when duties and demands often prevail, the thought of self-care may appear like a luxury, a reflection, or even a guilty pleasure. However, it is time to debunk these false assumptions and understand that self-care is not only a legitimate necessity but also a cornerstone of a healthy and satisfying existence. This chapter goes deeper into the crucial role of self-care, explaining why it is a critical factor in obtaining a dining a healthy weight and, more importantly, increasing your general well-being.

Definition of Self-Health:

Self-care is not just about indulgence or occasional attention; it is a multi-faceted strategy to sustain your mind, body, and spirit. It comprises a wide range of activities and practices that prioritize your health, pleasure, and inner serenity. Self-care is an act of compassion and self-respect, and it establishes the foundation on which you can build a rich life.

The Necessity of Self-Care for Weight Management:

Understanding the tremendous impact of self-care on your weight management journey is vital. Here is why self-care is not simply a luxury but a strategic and crucial component:

Stress Reduction: Chronic stress is a typical opponent in the fight against weight gain and obesity. High levels of stress stimulate the release of cortisol, a hormone that can lead to weight gain, especially in the abdomen area. Engaging in self-care techniques such as meditation, deep breathing, or spending time outside can greatly reduce stress levels, making it simpler to maintain a healthy weight.

Mental Health: Emotional eating that occurs during eating due to emotions other than hunger can be a serious impediment to successful weight loss.
You can manage emotional overeating via self-training, such as correspondence, counseling, or talking to a reliable friend.

Attentive Feeding: Self-health encourages and supports mindful eating. When you prioritize caring for yourself, you are more likely to eat intentionally and consciously, which makes it simpler for your body to identify and respond to symptoms of hunger and satiety. In turn, this promotes weight management.

Better Sleep: Quality sleep is a pillar of weight management. Self-care activities that promote optimal sleep hygiene, such as a relaxing ritual before bedtime, can increase sleep quality and support your weight objectives. Lack of sleep can influence hunger hormones and contribute to overeating.

Balanced Lifestyle: Self-health actively develops balance in your life. By taking time for activities that you genuinely enjoy, whether linked to relaxation, leisure, or social interaction, you are less likely to turn to food for comfort or entertainment.

Self-Compassion: Self-health increases self-compassion, lowering negative speech and self-criticism. This alteration in your inner dialogue can have a tremendous impact on your body image and overall well-being.

Incorporate Self-Care into Your Life:

Integrating self-care into your everyday life is not a hard endeavor, nor does it demand extra hours of effort. Rather, it is about making purposeful, aware choices that prioritize your well-being. Here's how to integrate self-care into your daily existence:

Identify Your Needs: Start by identifying which activities or routines resonate most with you and make you feel nourished and refreshed. These activities might vary significantly from person to person, ranging from simple pleasures such as reading a book to more demanding sports such as mountain trekking.

Plan it: Treat self-sufficiency with the same priority as work or other homework. Dedicate time to personal care chores by putting them in your daily or weekly calendar. This transforms self-care into non-negotiable commitments rather than optional indulgences.

Start Small: You don't need to commit hours of leisure time to self-health. Even a few minutes of deep breathing, a quick walk, or a moment of meditation can have a tangible difference. Starting simple and gradually improving your care routines assists you in forming lasting habits.

Make it a Habit: Consistency is the key to unlocking all the benefits of self-health. Incorporate self-care into your daily or weekly routine until it becomes a normal element of your life. The more consistent you are, the more you will feel the transformational impacts of self-care.

Learn to say no: An element of self-care is to set proper boundaries. It's the realization that you can't be everything for everyone all the time. Learning to say no when necessary allows you to put your well-being above excessive duties and please people.

Ask for Help: Self-care also requires requesting help when it is essential. Whether it's professional help from a therapist, mentor training, or just contacting friends and family for support, don't hesitate to seek aid while confronting hurdles. He's a potent sort of self-defense.

Self-Monitoring Beyond Physical Practices:

While self-health physical behaviors such as exercise and rest are vital, self-health extends beyond these areas. It comprises emotional care, which entails setting appropriate boundaries, controlling stress, and receiving support when needed. Mental care is engaging in things that engage your mind, such as reading, learning, or pursuing creative hobbies. Holistic self-care means achieving balance in all aspects of your lifegiving your relationships and alignment with your principles.

Adopt Self-Health as a Lifestyle:

After all, self-care is not a one-time effort or a periodic indulgence; it is a lifelong commitment to your well-being. It's about recognizing your intrinsic importance and taking proactive measures to take care of yourself, as you would for a loved one. By concentrating on self-care, you not only support your weight management goals but also generate a deeper sense of happiness and harmony in your life.

So, when you start evaluating self-wellness in this chapter, remember that it is not a luxury but an essential foundation of your health and enjoyment. Whether it's times of peaceful meditation, moments of delight, or moments of healing, self-care speaks to your commitment to leading a life that is not only existent but also prosperous. It is an assertion that you deserve to be fed, nourished, and valued, both by yourself and by the world around you.

Create a Long-Term Plan for Sustainable Results

In the pursuit of a better and more balanced existence, it is necessary to modify our thinking away from speedy healing and short-term transformations. The real key to success is establishing a long-term plan that not only helps you shed the additional pounds but also ensures that these benefits stand the test of time. This chapter takes a deep dive into the art and science of building a thorough long-term strategy — a plan that not only helps accomplish your weight management objectives but also allows you to maintain and cherish those results for years to come.

The Dangers of Short-Term Thinking:

In a society replete with promises of fast weight loss through crash diets and fashion regimens, it is crucial to recognize the traps of short-term thinking:

Fast Dieting: Fast-repair diets can lead to immediate weight loss, but they often finish with a painful cycle of fat loss and recovery known as yo-yo dieting. This trend not only has an impact on your physical health but can also affect your mental and emotional well-being.

Nutritional Deficiencies: Many extreme diets lack key nutrients. Although they can help you shed pounds rapidly, they can lead to long-term health problems owing to dietary shortages.

Non-Sustainable Behaviors: Extreme diets sometimes demand considerable alterations in eating habits that are difficult to maintain. When you ultimately revert to your regular dietary practices, the weight frequently returns as well.

Negative Relationship to Food: Restrictive diets can develop an unhealthy relationship with food, leading to feelings of guilt, anxiety, and even chaotic eating habits.

Components of a Long-Term Plan:

Developing a long-term plan for sustainable results is not a matter of deprivation, dramatic adjustments, or rigid timelines. Instead, it is about building healthy, sustainable practices that become organically an inherent part of your daily life. Here are the essential aspects of such a plan:

Set Reasonable Goals: Start by identifying reasonable and controllable goals. These objectives should be explicit, measurable, and timely. Rather than focusing on rapid weight loss, aim for a gradual and stable result that is more likely to endure.

Balanced Nutrition: Adopt a balanced approach to nutrition. Avoid excessive diets and focus on a well-rounded diet that comprises a variety of nutritional foods. Prioritize fruits, veggies, lean proteins, complete grains, and healthy fats.

Portion Control: Pay attention to portion dimensions. Learning to discern the proper portion sizes will help you balance calorie intake without feeling constrained.

Regular Physical Activity: Make regular activity part of your daily routine. Find pastimes that you genuinely love and make them a permanent presence in your life. Keep in mind that persistence matters more than intensity.

Eat Carefully: Cultivate careful eating habits. Watch out for symptoms of hunger and satiety, appreciate the tastes of your meals, and eat intentionally. This practice helps you build a healthier connection with food.

Support and Responsibility: Consider seeking support from a trained nutritionist, a fitness coach, or joining a weight loss club. Having someone to hold you accountable can provide valuable guidance and encouragement.

Lifestyle Changes: Focus on generating lasting alterations to the exercise mode. These could include planning meals, cooking more regularly at home, reducing sugary drinks, or finding healthier alternatives to beloved foods.

Stress Management: Implement stress management activities, such as meditation, deep breathing exercises, or yoga. Chronic stress can hinder weight loss efforts and undermine general well-being.

Sleep Optimization: Prioritize sleeping. Objective 7-9 hours of decent sleep per night. Inadequate sleep can influence appetite hormones and lead to weight gain.

Progress Tracking: Track your progress using a notebook or mobile app. Monitoring your nutrition, activities, and emotions can provide essential information and help you stay on track.

Flexibility and Adaptability: Understand that life is packed with unforeseen hurdles. Be adaptable and versatile in your weight management technique. If you face delays, do not perceive them as failures but as opportunities to learn and adjust.

The Mentality for Success:

Beyond the real components of a long-term plan, having the correct mindset is equally essential:

Patience: Recognize that sustainable weight loss takes time. Avoid the appeal of rapid corrections and remain patient and dedicated to your objective.

Self-Compassion: Practice kindness for oneself. Be kind to yourself, especially in times of difficulty or disappointment. Weight management is not a linear process, and treating yourself with compassion can enhance your resilience.

Positive Self-Talk: Challenge negative self-talk and establish a positive inner conversation. Focus on your accomplishments and progress, whatever their scale.

Resilience: develop resilience to adversity. Understand that chess is inherent in every path, and it does not define your ultimate aim.

Adopt Everlasting Health:

Creating a long-term plan for lasting results is not about hitting a specific number on the scale; it is about embracing a life of health, vitality, and well-being. It's about feeding your body, mind, and spirit with love and care, and it's a dedication to a journey that goes well beyond weight reduction. By adopting healthy and sustainable behaviors and encouraging the proper mindset, you may accomplish weight management objectives and ensure that these benefits are not merely ephemeral, but a lasting monument to your dedication to a healthier, happier you.

As you read this chapter, remember that your journey to sustainable success is not a race but a lifelong adventure. It is an examination of self-discovery, self-improvement, and self-care. By designing a strategy that stresses your well-being and sustainability, you are placing yourself on the path not only to achieve your goals but also to thrive in the magnificent tapestry of life itself.

Chapter 5: Sustainable weight Loss Strategies: Achieving Sustainable Results

Are you tired of the unending cycle of diets that promise instant solutions but leave you feeling unfulfilled and discouraged? It's time to focus your attention on sustainable weight-loss strategies that not only help you lose pounds but also allow you to maintain a healthier lifestyle in the long run. But let's look at some behaviors that we need to get rid of to reach our weight target. Let's examine these methods in greater detail:

Break the Habit of Being Overweight

Breaking the habit of being overweight involves a complicated approach anchored in self-awareness and determination:

Self-Reflection: Start by truly thinking about your present behaviors and how they led to your weight. Recognize emotional eating behaviors, sedentary activities, and any unhealthy link with food. Understanding the fundamental reasons for these habits is the cornerstone of change.

Set Clear Goals: Set specific and measurable weight-loss goals. Rather than vague objectives, establish precise targets, such as losing a certain quantity of pounds or inches within a specified timeframe. Break down these long-term goals into smaller, manageable actions to track your progress efficiently.

Eat Carefully: Adopt careful eating habits. This means activating all your senses when you eat, enjoying every item, and reducing distractions during meals. Eating mindfully helps you become more aware of your eating patterns, helping you recognize and modify the behaviors that contribute to overeating.

Create a Support System: Share your weight loss objectives with friends, and family, or join a support group. Having a support system offers encouragement, responsibility, and a sense of community throughout your journey. It is a reminder that you are not alone in your search for a healthy life.

Replace Negative Self-Speaking: Challenge and rearrange negative self-speaking and restrict notions about your abilities to lose weight. Replace these thoughts with affirmations that promote your confidence and commitment to change. Cultivating a growth mentality is key because it helps you perceive obstacles as opportunities for advancement.

Selling on Weight Loss

Selling yourself on weight loss is about motivating and convincing you that the approach is useful and feasible.

Visualize Success: Create a clear mental picture of your desired weight, health, and lifestyle. Imagine engaging in activities you love, feeling confident, and enjoying increased well-being. Visualizing achievement makes your goals more tangible and achievable.

Track Progress: Keep a detailed record of your successes. Document your weight loss progress with journals, photographs, or specialist monitoring applications. Celebrate every triumph, no matter how tiny, to boost your drive to improve and remind you of your progress.

Educate Yourself: Invest time in learning the benefits of weight loss beyond appearances. Understanding how reducing excess weight can improve your general health, raise energy levels, lessen the risk of chronic illness, and improve your quality of life Knowledge is a powerful motivator.

Set Prices: Establish a price scheme for your weight reduction goals. Designate meaningful, non-nutritional rewards for certain steps. Whether it's a spa day, a new item of clothing, or a weekend getaway, these prizes serve as positive reinforcement for your achievements.

Surround Yourself with Optimism: Make sure your environment is full of happiness and inspiration. Follow social media profiles, read books, and research articles that encourage healthy lifestyle advice and weight loss success stories.

Surrounding yourself with optimism enhances your motivation.

Search for Professional Orientation: Consider visiting a certified dietitian or a fitness professional for specialist help. They can help you build a tailored plan that focuses on your unique requirements and obstacles, which dramatically boosts your chances of success.

Practice Self-Compassion: Recognize that reverses are an intrinsic element of any journey of development. Instead of reprimanding yourself for temporary failures, cultivate compassion for yourself. Treat yourself with care and forgiveness, recognizing that your commitment to long-term improvement is what is really important.

Breaking the habit of being overweight and persuading yourself to embrace weight loss is a fundamental transition that takes a mix of self-awareness, realistic objectives, positive reinforcement, and a tireless drive to sustain change. By immersing yourself in these attitude adjustments and practices, you are establishing the basis for a happier and more fulfilling life.

Let's Examine These Methods in Greater Detail:

1. Eat Carefully: Sustainable weight loss begins with full consciousness. Instead of rushing your food, take the time to taste your food rather than eating quickly or mindlessly.

Instead of rushing into meals or eating without purpose, take the time to savor your food. Engage your senses by exploring flavors, textures, and fragrances. By being completely present throughout meals, you will become more familiar with your body's hunger and indicators of satiety, leading to improved portion control and wiser food choices.

2. Balanced Nutrition: Adopt a balanced approach to nutrition. Abandon the idea of rigid diets that omit whole food groupings. Instead, prefer a diet rich in fruits, vegetables, lean protein, whole grains, and healthy fats. These foods supply the required nutrition and lasting energy, keeping you happy and nourished.

3. Portion Control: Learning to detect the appropriate portion quantities is vital. Be careful with portion sizes and avoid trying to oversize your meals. Using smaller dishes and utensils might help you naturally reduce portion size, limiting overfeeding without feeling deprived.

4. Regular Physical Activity: Incorporate regular physical activity into your diet. Find delightful forms of exercise, be it dancing, hiking, swimming, or just taking quick walks. Physical activity not only burns calories, but also stimulates metabolism, enhances muscle tone, and improves general well-being.

5. Self-Reflection: Dive deep into self-reflection. Explore the emotional and psychological components that can contribute to your weight concerns. Establish healthy management strategies to replace these behaviors by identifying the triggers of emotional feeding, emotional eating, or irresponsible snacking.

6. Assistance System: Seek aid from friends, family, or a weight loss club. Sharing your path with others gives you encouragement and responsibility. Having a support system can make the difference between giving up and persevering towards your goals.

7. Slow and Stable Progress: Understand that lasting weight loss is a protracted process. Rather than seeking fast revolutions, focus on incremental, consistent adjustments over time. Celebrate every step of the trip to stay motivated.

8. Education and Awareness-Raising: Educate yourself on the benefits of sustainable weight loss. Beyond aesthetics, decreasing excess weight can reduce the risk of chronic diseases, raise energy levels, and improve overall health. Knowing these long-term gains could encourage your dedication.

9. Self-Compassion: Be compassionate to yourself during your weight loss journey. Avoid self-criticism and cultivate self-compassion. Understand that delays are natural and provide opportunities for learning and advancement.

10. Long-Term Perspective: alter your thinking from aiming for short-term results to adopting a lifelong commitment to health and well-being. Durable weight loss is not about transient treatments but about creating persistent behaviors that support a healthier you.

These sustainable weight-loss strategies do not rely on restrictive diets or quick treatments. It is about building a healthy, aware connection with food, supporting your body with nutritional choices, and adopting a lifestyle that generates lasting benefits. Remember, your path is unique, and the key to success is to select the solutions that work best for you and connect with your own goals and preferences. So, go on this journey with confidence, knowing that sustainable weight loss is within your reach, and lasting results await your efforts.

Integrate Physical Activity into Your Routine: The Secret to a Healthier You

Are you ready to advance your path toward a better lifestyle? Incorporating physical activity into your daily routine is a revolutionary trend that not only improves weight loss but also contributes to your general well-being. Let us examine this subject in full, with clear, pleasant, and actionable ideas:

1. Locate what you Like: The first step to making physical activity a constant part of your life is to locate activities that you genuinely enjoy. It can be dancing, cycling, swimming, hiking, or even a simple walk in the park. When you wait for your hobbies, being active becomes a pleasure, not a duty.

2. Start Gently and Gradually: If you are new to regular exercise, remember that little steps lead to major changes. Start with basic goals, such as a 15-minute walk every day or a short home workout. As your endurance and confidence build, you can gradually increase the duration and intensity of your activities.

3. Set Realistic Goals: Determining feasible goals is crucial to motivation. Rather than aiming to make a major change overnight, set modest, attainable targets. Celebrate every stride, whether it's running your first mile or making a new yoga pose.

4. Create an Arrangement: Just like you manage meals and work meetings, devote time for physical activity in your daily routine. Treat your workouts like appointments you can't skip. Consistency is the key to reaping the advantages of physical activity.

5. Mix It Up: Variety is not only the spice of life but also the key to maintaining inspiration in your fitness program. Incorporate numerous types of exercises throughout the week to engage various muscle groups and minimize boredom.

6. Accompanying System: Consider finding an exercise companion or joining group fitness programs. Having someone to practice with can make the process more pleasurable and ensure responsibility. It is also a good opportunity to interact while being active.

7. Listen to your Body: Pay heed to your body's signals. If you are fatigued or hurt, it is excellent to take a day off or partake in lighter workouts such as stretching or yoga. Rest and recovery are vital parts of a healthy workout plan.

8. Stay Hydrated: Remember to stay hydrated before, during, and after your workouts. Water helps your body function during exercise and helps in recovery.

9. Monitor Progress: Follow your progress to stay motivated. Consider using fitness apps or portable gadgets to log your workouts, steps, or heart rate. Following your accomplishments can be encouraging and help you create new goals.

10. Embrace Coherence: cohesion is the secret sauce of long-term success. Regular physical activity not only helps eliminate excess weight, but also improves cardiovascular health, strengthens muscles, speeds up metabolism, and elevates your mood.

11. Make it a Diary: Instead of treating physical activity as a transient activity, aim to make it an inherent part of your everyday life. When exercise becomes a habit, you will reap the rewards of enhanced health and vigor for years to come.

Incorporating physical activity into your daily routine is not just about losing weight; it is about having a better, more vibrant existence. By choosing the things you like, setting fair goals, and making exercise a continuous part of your routine, you invest not just in your physical health, but also in your mental and emotional well-being. So, toss away your socks, go to bed, and leave the way to health that you're starting. Your body and mind will thank you.

Understanding the Value of Self-Care: Cultivating your Well-being

In participating in modern life, it's easy to forget a critical element of your entire health—self-wellness. Far from being a luxury, self-care is a vital activity that plays a key role in your physical, emotional, and mental well-being. Let's investigate the relevance of self-care with clarity, empathy, and practical knowledge:

1. Self-Monitoring Defined

Self-care is more than simply bubble baths and spa days; it comprises any purposeful effort made to preserve or improve your health. This encompasses physical self-care (exercise and nutrition), emotional self-health (stress management and self-compassion), and mental self-help (mindfulness and relaxation).

2. Fill in your Reservations

Think of taking care of yourself as well as recharging your internal supplies. Just as a car needs gas to run, you need self-care to retain your vigor and resilience. Failing to take care of oneself can lead to weariness, stress, and a compromised immune system.

3. Prioritize Physical Health

Self-care begins with your physical well-being. Regular exercise, a balanced diet, and proper sleep are key components. These actions not only improve your physique but also increase your mood and cognitive performance.

4. Emotional Well-Being

Emotional self-care entails identifying and managing stress, practicing self-compassion, and engaging in activities that offer joy. It is about acknowledging your feelings and finding suitable strategies to handle them.

5. Mental Well-Being

Mental self-sufficiency focuses on feeding your intellect. It requires exercising full consciousness, engaging in things that interest your intellect, and making sure you have free time to unwind. A properly rested mind is more creative, concentrated, and resilient.

6. Boundaries

Setting adequate limits is a sort of self-care. Learn to say no when required, convey your demands effectively, and avoid being too invested. Limits save you time and energy.

7. Stress Reduction

Chronic stress can affect your health. Prioritize stress reduction practices such as deep breathing, meditation, yoga, or spending time outside. Stress management is a key element of self-care.

8. Self-Compassion

Treat yourself with care and understanding. Replace self-criticism with compassion. Understand that it is okay to make mistakes or to have delays; it is a part of the human being.

9. Prevention

Do not cure: Self-health is a sort of preventive medicine. By taking proactive care of oneself, you lessen the likelihood of physical and mental health problems. Prevention is often more beneficial than treatment.

10. A customized Strategy

Self-care is very personal. What seems to work for a certain individual could be less helpful for another. Make an effort try numerous self-health strategies to discover what's effective for you and fits into your everyday routine.

11. No Remorse: Being self-aware is not being selfish

It is necessary. You shouldn't feel bad for taking the time to care for yourself. You are better able to take care of people and carry out your obligations when you put your needs first.

12. Issues Linked to Coherence

Self-care is not a one-time event but a lifelong discipline. Consistency is required to gain from it. Incorporate self-care into your daily, weekly, and monthly regimen.

13. Request Assistance

If self-care is tough, try to acquire the support of a therapist, a counselor, or a support group. They can provide information and ideas for efficiently applying self-care.

14. Improving Physical Health

Exercise consistently, a component of self-care, not only promotes weight management but also enhances your muscles and bones.

A proper diet, another aspect of self-health, ensures that your body receives critical nutrients for optimal functioning.

Adequate sleep, often disregarded in our busy lives, is crucial for physical recovery, immune system support, and hormonal balance.

15. Improved Mental Clarity

Self-care practices such as mindfulness meditation and relaxation techniques promote mental clarity by decreasing mental illnesses and increasing focused thought.

A clear mind is better adapted to dealing with demanding activities and making educated judgments, whether at work or in personal life.

16. Increased Emotional Resilience

Self-care increases emotional resilience by offering techniques to cope with stress, anxiety, and negative feelings.

Regular compassion and contemplation can lead to stronger emotional regulation and an enhanced ability to go back after failure.

17. Improving Relations

The benefits of self-sufficiency extend to your relationships. When you are emotionally balanced and less stressed, you can communicate more effectively and satisfy the demands of loved ones.

You will also be less inclined to rely on people for your emotional well-being, easing the burden on relationships.

18. Increased Productivity

Contrary to the assumption that self-care takes time, it actually boosts productivity. Taking breaks, remaining well rested, and minimizing stress assist in enhancing production levels.

When you focus on caring for yourself, you are more likely to prevent weariness, which leads to long-term sustainable production.

19. Increased Creativity

Personal care activities like exploring new interests or just having time to dream might increase your creativity.

Creativity can lead to inventive problem-solving and a new perspective on life's difficulties.

20. Stress Reduction

Chronic stress impacts your physical and emotional well-being. Self-care strategies, such as deep breathing exercises, progressive muscular relaxation, or even spending time in nature,

Reduce the release of stress hormones such as cortisol.

This leads to a more tranquil and balanced state of mind, lowering the chance of stress-related health problems.

21. Improving Self-Esteem

Engaging in self-care sends a powerful message to yourself that you deserve love and attention. It supports self-esteem and can lead to greater self-worth.

This increased self-esteem can have a favorable effect on your relationships, your profession, and the overall pleasure of life.

22. Lifelong Learning

Self-care often includes things that strengthen your intellect, such as reading, taking classes, or learning new abilities.

Lifelong learning not only keeps your mind fresh but also delivers a sense of accomplishment and personal progress.

23. Get rid of Digital Overload

The constant connection of the digital era can lead to overload and weariness of information. Self-care includes setting limits on technology and taking regular breaks.

These intervals allow you to detach, recharge, and reconnect with the real world, which decreases the detrimental consequences of using screens.

24. Role Modeling

Practicing self-care sets an example for everyone around you, especially if you have children. You exemplify the significance of self-care and inspire others to prioritize it.

By modeling self-health, you generate a ripple effect of well-being in your community.

25. Long-Term Happiness

Ultimately, self-care adds to long-term happiness and life satisfaction. It is about building a worldwide sense of well-being that goes beyond transient pleasure.

By making self-care a priority, you invest in your future happiness and general quality of life.

Self-care is not a luxury; it is necessary for a well-balanced and meaningful life. It is about finding harmony in all areas of your well-being - physical, emotional, and mental—and making sure you have the tools and resilience to transcend the heights and downs of life with grace and enthusiasm.

Create a Long-Term Plan for Sustainable Results: Your Roadmap to Sustainable Wellness

As you pursue your road toward sustained well-being and positive development, it is vital to build a clear and complete long-term plan. This plan will act as your guide, guiding you through the ups and downs of your health and lifestyle improvement. Let us explore this subject with clarity, sensitivity, and operational knowledge:

1. Define your Vision

Take the time to eloquently define your vision of your well-being. What does it look like when you have achieved your goals? Does he experience greater vitality, adjust vto his preferred attire, or have the perseverance to follow his passions? Your vision should inspire and encourage you.

2. Define SMART Objectives

Break down your vision into precise, measurable, attainable, relevant, and temporary goals (SMART). For example, instead of expressing "I want to lose weight", do it specifically: "I aim to lose 20 pounds in six months by following a balanced diet and exercising regularly."

3. Break it Down

Split your SMART goals into smaller, more manageable tasks. For example, if your aim is to run a marathon, start with a strategy to run shorter distances and progressively increase your mileage. Celebrate every stage of the journey.

4. Prioritize Habits

Identify the important habits that will support your ambitions. These may include: eating carefully, appreciating every bite, and picking foods rich in nutrition.

Incorporate at least 30 minutes of physical activity into your day, whether walking, dancing, or hitting the gym.

Practice stress management strategies such as yoga, meditation, or journalism.

Make sure you receive 7-9 hours of great sleep every night.

5. Sustainable Nutrition

Focus on creating a lasting relationship with food. This means avoiding sudden dieting and instead making wiser and steady decisions. Include extra fruit, vegetables, whole grains, lean meats, and healthy fats in your diet.

6. Constant Physical Activity

Commit yourself to regular exercise that you like. This could be dancing, hiking, swimming, or any activity that keeps you moving. Consistency in exercise is more important than intensity.

7. Careful Stress Management

Develop a directory of stress management methods that work for you. This could include deep breathing techniques, progressive muscle relaxation, or simply spending time outdoors. Regular stress management is key to preserving your well-being.

8. Social Support

Share your goals with your friends, family, or a support group. Having a support network brings encouragement and responsibility. It's good to know that you're not alone on this road.

9. Ongoing Education

Keep an open mind and a curious spirit. The health and wellness industry is evolving. Keep up on the most recent developments in science, fashion, and wellness strategies. You can choose wisely with the help of this information.

10. Review and Modification

Keep a close eye on your development. Are your goals being met on schedule? If not, don't be disheartened; take use of these opportunities for reflection and adaptation. As you change, your plan should too.

11. Self-Compassion

Self-compassion is a key component of your journey. Remember that perfection is not the aim, it is development. Be kind to yourself, especially after chess. Learn from these moments and continue on.

12. Celebrate Success

Recognize and appreciate your achievements. Whether it's completing a key milestone in weight loss, running a mile quicker, or reducing stress, these celebrations boost your commitment and improve your motivation.

13. Ask for Professional Guidance

If you face problems or need particular counsel, try seeing health specialists or nutrition and exercise experts. They can provide knowledgeable guidance and recommendations depending on your individual needs.

14. Long-Term Perspectives

Keep the image in mind. Sustainable well-being is about creating a balanced, sustainable lifestyle that promotes your health and happiness throughout your life. Adopt the mentality that the trip itself is as essential as the destination.

Creating a long-term plan for sustainable results is a dynamic and transforming process. It is about making mindful decisions every day that meet your vision of well-being. By setting SMART goals, cultivating healthy habits, seeking support when needed, and remaining fit, you build a foundation for a better, fuller life, one step at a time. Your journey is a monument to your commitment to self-improvement and your trust in a greater and healthier future.

Final thoughts: a road map for sustainable well-being

"Nourish Your Way to a Healthy Weight: Embrace Food, Trust Your Body, and Get Lasting Results" is not just a book; it's a road to everlasting well-being. It acts as a beneficial companion on your journey to a healthier, more dynamic being, delivering in-depth knowledge and practical assistance.

In a society overloaded with diets and quick fixes, this book stands out as a beacon of wisdom and direction. He understands that obtaining a dining a healthy weight is not a single activity. Instead, it embraces the complexity of human well-being, addressing not only the bodily components but also the emotional, mental, and social components of our existence.

The width of the book on the subject and its real-world applicability make it a fantastic resource for anyone striving for actual transformation. It goes beyond the seeming promise of speedy weight loss and plunges deep into the psychology of eating, the power of self-compassion, and the advantages of full consciousness. It educates readers about the advantages of shifting away from restrictive diets and developing a balanced and flexible attitude toward food.

In addition, the book teaches readers the knowledge needed to spot recurrent tendencies that often contribute to overeating and overweight. It provides individuals with strategies to refocus their cognitive processes, providing a basis for sustainable change. It is not just about losing weight; it will be about breaking the habits that no longer serve you and building new, healthy ones.

The chapters on self-care and physical activity underscore the general character of well-being. They recognize that health goes beyond the plate and extends to our everyday routines and self-compassion practices. The book teaches readers the various benefits acquired from regular physical activity, emphasizing that exercise is not only a weight management tool but a key component of mental and emotional well-being.

Finally, the book's counsel on building a long-term plan for sustainable effects demonstrates its commitment to offering readers the skills they need to support their development. He realizes that meaningful transformation takes time and entails adaptability. It empowers readers to establish meaningful objectives, prioritize healthy behaviors, and approach their journey of well-being with a feeling of purpose and resolve.

In conclusion, "Nourish Your Way to a Healthy Weight" is more than a book; it's a thorough educational journey that gives you the information and knowledge you need to alter your life. It is a strategy for permanent well-being, leading you to a better, happier, and more fulfilling future. As you undertake this transforming journey, remember that the lessons of the book are not just words on pages, but a means of genuine and enduring change. Embrace information, apply it to your life, and allow it to be your compass on the way to the best version of yourself.

Reader's Digest

Here's a job for you: Adjust your love for food with controlled weight reduction

Congratulations on your commitment to a healthier life! Keep in mind that your procedure does not need to be about difficulties; adjust to thoughtful judgments that meet your aims while enjoying the range of foods you adore. Here's your school work as a tutor to guide you towards sustainable weight loss without giving in to your number one extravagance:

1. Arrangement of a Thoughtful Dinner:

Look for the meal arrangement that consolidates your number one food variety while retaining a balance. Explicit indications of the days or occasions when you can benefit from these irreproachable remedies. Combine them with complimentary heavier dinners to produce a fair dish.

2. Fragment Control: Practice fragment control to see the benefit of your food assortments without revealing them. Use more subtle dishes, bowls, and plates to help regulate your pieces. Enjoy each nibble, and take as much time as planned to thoroughly indulge in the flavors.

3. Eat with Caution: Practice a deliberate diet based on signs of desire and integrity. Before beginning with your number one treatment, make sure you are extremely energetic. Eat gradually, participate in each snack, and stop when you are effortless.

4. Consolidate the Thick Food Sources of the Supplement: Make the additional thick food variety a constant in your diet regimen. These dietary sources supply necessary vitamins, enhance your well-being, and make you feel full. Incorporate a mix of organic goods, veggies, lean proteins, nutritious grains, and solid fats into your dinners.

5. Hydration Issues: Stay hydrated by drinking plenty of water throughout the day. In some instances, what we assume to be appetite is really thirst. Focus on water, natural teas, and other moisturizing drinks to assist your body's needs.

6. Regular Active Job: Participate in the regular practical work you like. Whether jogging, walking, swimming, or performing yoga, find exercises that complement your inclinations. Real working weight loss also adds to your entire well-being.

7. Balance of Practice: Remember that balance is key. It's wonderful to engage in your #1 meal types every time so often, although watch out for section sizes and recurrence. Balance is crucial for successful weight loss.

8. Implement Realistic Objectives: Set acceptable and achievable goals for your weight reduction business. Focus on progress rather than perfection. Celebrate even modest victories and keep an eye on your growth to stay encouraged.

9. Log of Your Decisions: Keep a food notebook where you document your dinners, tastes, and joys. This can help you keep track of your judgments, find examples, and make changes on a case-by-case basis.

10. Seeking Help:

Interface with an emotionally valuable network that energizes your path. Whether it's friends, relatives, or online networks, discussing your meetings and concerns can provide you encouragement and responsibility.

Let us renew our stories, put the emphasis on trust, and praise the tiny wins that create our approach.

As you read through these pages, let the wisdom found there serve as your compass. Accept the adventure it offers—one that unites the body, brain, and mind—in its entirety. May you go on your trip with a sense of self-assurance and a fresh-found awe for life's fine needlework. Never forget that living a healthy, prosperous, and full life involves many different factors in addition to losing weight. The procedure for discovery is as follows:

A Practical Work Schedule

Your Road to Reasonable Change: The Complete Guide to Weight Loss

Good luck on your quest for success and permanent weight loss! This instruction book intends to give you important, observable, and trustworthy breakthroughs. Each business was established to assist you in living a healthy lifestyle without having to give up the meals you like.

Week 1: Take Everything in

Task 1: For several weeks, record your eating habits. Record your joys, snacks, and celebrations, as well as your emotions and level of passion.

Task 2: Determine your preferred dietary preferences and the types of foods you most enjoy eating. Note how frequently you drink them.

Week 2: Modified the Time for Dinner

Task 1: Plan your dinners for the next seven days, including a variety of supplements in addition to your main food source.

Task 2: Schedule certain days or times to moderately use your preferred traits.

Week 3: Mindful Eating Routines

Task 1: Work without interruption while eating comes first. Take into account the taste, look, and aroma of each mastic.

Task 2: Use the desired completion scale (1–10) to rate your hunger at dinner. When you're genuinely upset, plan your meals and stop when you're full.

Week four: A Partial Examination

Task 1: Arrange the components on smaller plates and in a bowl to change the size of the segments.

Task 2: To preserve the tastes without removing them, bake them in manageable pieces while consuming your favorite candy.

Week 5: Hydration and Development

Task 1: Consume at least eight glasses of water per day to stay hydrated.

Task 2: Decide on a worthwhile, sincere endeavor that you can manage on several occasions this week.

Week 6: Progress Monitoring and Evaluation

Task 1: Think about your adventure so far. Has anything changed about your eating habits, energy level, or prospects?

Task 2: Track your actual progress in Task 2 by taking measurements or photos. You should be proud of whatever development you see.

Week 7: Modified Choices

Task 1: Individualized dinners with a balance of veggies, complete grains, lean protein, and healthy fats should be offered.

Task 2: While incorporating your favorite indulgence into your weekly strategy, emphasize how your choices complement one another.

Week 8: Reflection and Confidence

Task 1: Practice making affirmations that are supportive of your desire to reduce weight and boost your self-esteem.

Task 2: Envision yourself leading a better, happier life. Imagine enjoying your favorite meal in moderation while being mindful of your budget.

Week 9: Seek Out Assistance

Task 1: Involves talking about your weight-loss goals with a partner or parent. Ask for their comfort and support.

Task 2: Take part in a conversation about a related subject in a group setting, either locally or online. Christmas Week

Week 10: Rejoicing and Reflection

Task 1: Recognize your success thus far! Treating yourself will allow you to enjoy a non-food reward for your devotion.

Task 2: Consider your earlier experiences. What new insights did you get into your character, routines, and relationship with food?

Please note that this is informational advice rather than a rigid schedule. Your obligations should reflect your interests and way of life. The objective is to promote useful behaviors that align with your path to success on a global scale. Maintain your diligence, look after yourself, and be mindful of your development as you go.

You can also check this out:

Here is a superb weekly work schedule that fulfills the requirements of this technique and results in substantial breakthroughs to help you incorporate these ideas into your daily practice:

Week 1: Start off Slowly.

Concentrating on full consciousness, Resolve to keep an objective eye on your food habits this week. Keep an eye on your favorite food groups and the times of day you tend to overeat.

Week 2: Different Dinners

Favorite food choices Reconciliation: Create events that feature your preferred food groups. Combine them with vegetables, lean protein, and grain-rich foods for a stunning and nutrient-dense feast.

Week 3: Body Association

Always pay heed to your body's instincts when eating intuitively. Ask yourself if you are anxious before eating, then ey6yat until you are truly full.

Week 4: More Happiness

Look for pleasant exercises and, during the process, numerous proactive roles. At least 30 minutes should be dedicated to something you truly enjoy doing each day.

Week 5: Emphasize Drinking Water

Keep hydrated: Always carry a bottle of water with you, and make an effort to drink about eight glasses of water each day.

Week 6: Success Possibilities

Affirmations and gratitude: To start the day off right, make a list of three things you are grateful for.

Week 7: Refrain from Being Indulgent

Control practice: Choose your therapy's first participation day with care. Reli finished every bite and showed up there on time.

Week 8: Appreciating Your Body Body Love:

When you look in the mirror each day, pay attention to one feature of your body that you love.

Week 9: Progress Assessment

extraordinary successes Think about whether you feel less focused, more lively, or upbeat. Respect their achievements.

Week 10: A Variety of Ways of Living

Daily routine: Incorporate a cautious diet and ecstatic growth into your schedule. Keep these tactics in mind as you go about your daily activities.

You must understand that consistency is crucial. Approach each week with a positive attitude and the resolve to implement minor changes. A manner of living that capitalizes on your assets and fosters prosperity is the aim. As you move forward with this plan, you'll typically end up adopting more cutting-edge trends and achieving your weight-loss goals while participating in activities you enjoy.

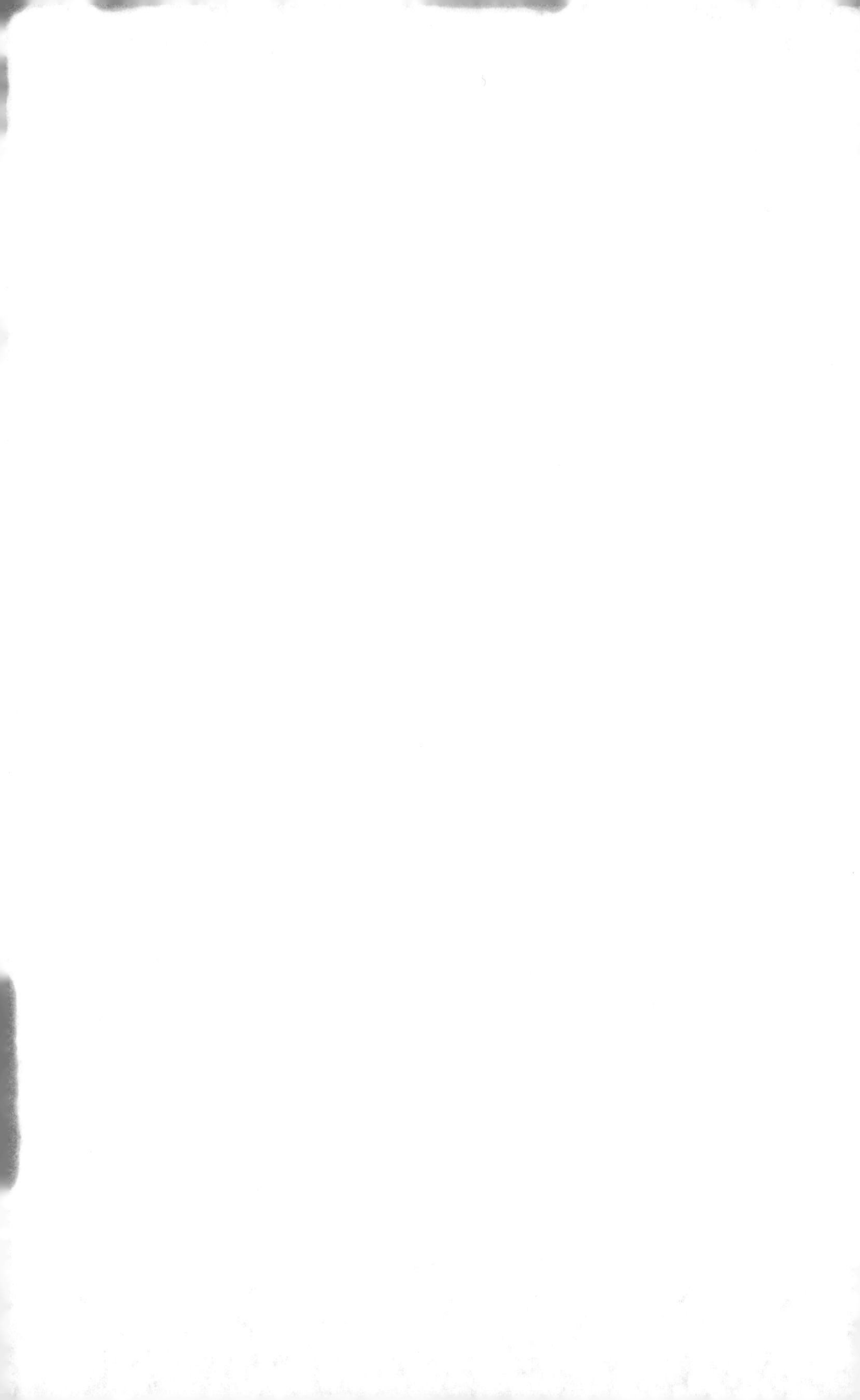